A COMPREHENSIVE GUIDE TO REVERSING OSTEOPOROSIS

Diet, workout and natural remedies for stronger bones without medications

Frank Cooks

Copyright © 2024 by Frank Cooks

Table of Contents

A COMPREHENSIVE GUIDE TO REVERSING OSTEOPOROSIS — **1**

Introduction — **6**

Chapter 1: Understanding Osteoporosis — **14**

Definition and Causes: — 17

Risk Factors: — 21

Impact on Quality of Life: — 24

Chapter 2: Diagnosis and Assessment — **30**

Bone Density Testing: — 33

Fracture Risk Assessment — 36

Laboratory Tests for Bone Health: — 41

Part I: Dietary Strategies — 44

Chapter 3: Essential Nutrients for Bone Health — **50**

Calcium Sources and Requirements: — 54

Vitamin D and Sunlight Exposure: — 58

Magnesium, Vitamin K, and Other Key Nutrients: — 63

Chapter 4: Foods to Include and Avoid — **68**

Bone-Friendly Foods: — 72

Foods That Weaken Bones: — 77

Importance of a Balanced Diet: — 81

Part II: Exercise and Physical Activity — 85

Chapter 5: Importance of Physical Activity — **90**

Weight-Bearing Exercises: — 94

Resistance Training for Bone Strength: — 98

Flexibility and Balance Exercises: 104

Chapter 6: Tailored Workout Plans   110

Beginner's Exercise Routine: 114

Incorporating Exercise into Daily Life: 123

Part III: Natural Remedies: 128

Chapter 7: Herbal and Nutritional Supplements 134

Benefits of Herbal Remedies: 138

Supplementing Calcium and Vitamin D: 142

Safety and Precautions: 147

Chapter 8: Lifestyle Modifications   152

Stress Reduction Techniques: 156

Smoking and Alcohol Cessation: 159

Sleep and Bone Health: 163

Part IV: Bonus - Healthy Bone Recipes   167

Chapter 9: Nutritious Recipes for Stronger Bones   172

Breakfast Ideas: 176

Lunch and Dinner Recipes: 179

Snacks and Beverages: 184

Conclusion   190

Introduction

Once upon a time in a small town nestled amidst rolling hills, there lived an elderly woman named Mrs. Thompson. She had always been an active and vibrant soul, but as the years went by, osteoporosis began to take its toll on her bones. Fractures became frequent, and Mrs. Thompson found herself struggling with daily tasks she once took for granted.

One day, while browsing the local library, Mrs. Thompson stumbled upon a book titled "The Complete Guide to Reversing Osteoporosis." Intrigued, she checked it out and began reading it with a newfound determination.

The book was a treasure trove of knowledge, filled with dietary tips, exercise routines, natural remedies, and inspiring stories of individuals who had successfully reversed osteoporosis. Mrs. Thompson immersed herself in the book, taking notes, highlighting key points, and slowly implementing the recommended changes into her life.

She started incorporating more calcium-rich foods like leafy greens, dairy products, and fortified cereals into her diet. Vitamin D became her best friend, as she soaked up the sun's rays during morning walks. The book guided her through gentle yet effective exercises that strengthened her bones and improved her balance.

Months passed, and Mrs. Thompson's dedication began to yield results. She felt stronger, more energetic, and her fractures became less frequent. Her doctor was amazed at her progress during regular check-ups.

But it wasn't just about physical changes; the book had also inspired Mrs. Thompson mentally and emotionally. She embraced a positive mindset, believing wholeheartedly that she could win the battle against osteoporosis.

One sunny afternoon, Mrs. Thompson climbed to the top of a hill overlooking her town. With a heart full of gratitude, she breathed in the fresh air and marveled at the beauty around her. She knew that her journey wasn't over, but she also knew that she had the knowledge and determination to continue living a fulfilling life despite osteoporosis.

As she stood there, a gentle breeze ruffled her hair, and she whispered to herself, "Thank you, book, for showing me that with perseverance and knowledge, even the toughest battles can be won." And with that, Mrs. Thompson descended the hill, ready to face each day with renewed strength and hope.

Welcome to "The Complete Guide to Reversing Osteoporosis," a comprehensive manual designed to empower you on your journey towards stronger, healthier bones. Osteoporosis, a condition characterized by weakening of the bones, affects millions of individuals worldwide, particularly the elderly and postmenopausal women. While osteoporosis may seem daunting, this book is your roadmap to understanding, managing, and ultimately reversing this condition.

In these pages, you will embark on a transformative exploration of osteoporosis, delving into its causes, risk factors, and the profound impact it can have on your quality of life. But more importantly, you will discover practical strategies, backed by scientific research, to not only halt the progression of osteoporosis but also to reverse its effects and regain bone strength.

Our journey begins with a comprehensive overview of osteoporosis, unraveling its complexities and shedding light on the intricate interplay between bone health, nutrition, exercise, and lifestyle. You will gain insights into the importance of bone density testing, fracture risk assessment, and laboratory evaluations, empowering you to take proactive steps in managing your bone health.

Part I of this guide focuses on dietary strategies, unveiling the vital nutrients essential for bone strength and resilience. From calcium and vitamin D to magnesium, vitamin K, and beyond, you will discover the optimal sources and recommended intake levels of these nutrients, alongside practical tips on incorporating bone-friendly foods into your daily meals.

In Part II, we delve into the realm of exercise and physical activity, exploring the pivotal role of weight-bearing exercises, resistance training, flexibility routines, and balance exercises in enhancing bone density and muscle strength. Tailored workout plans cater to individuals of all fitness levels, ensuring that everyone can embark on a journey towards stronger bones.

Part III is dedicated to natural remedies, where you will explore the potential benefits of herbal supplements, nutritional interventions, and lifestyle modifications in promoting bone health. You will learn how to harness the healing power of nature while adopting habits that support overall well-being.

As a bonus, Part IV presents a collection of healthy bone recipes, carefully crafted to nourish your body with the essential nutrients needed for optimal bone health. From breakfast delights to savory dinners and nutritious snacks, these recipes will inspire you to embrace a bone-friendly culinary journey.

Throughout this guide, you will encounter real-life success stories, expert insights, and practical tips that bridge the gap between knowledge and action. Whether you are seeking to prevent osteoporosis, manage its symptoms, or reverse its effects, this book equips you with the tools, strategies, and motivation to reclaim your bone health and vitality.

Are you ready to embark on a transformative journey towards osteoporosis reversal? Let's dive in and empower ourselves to build stronger bones, healthier lives, and a brighter future.

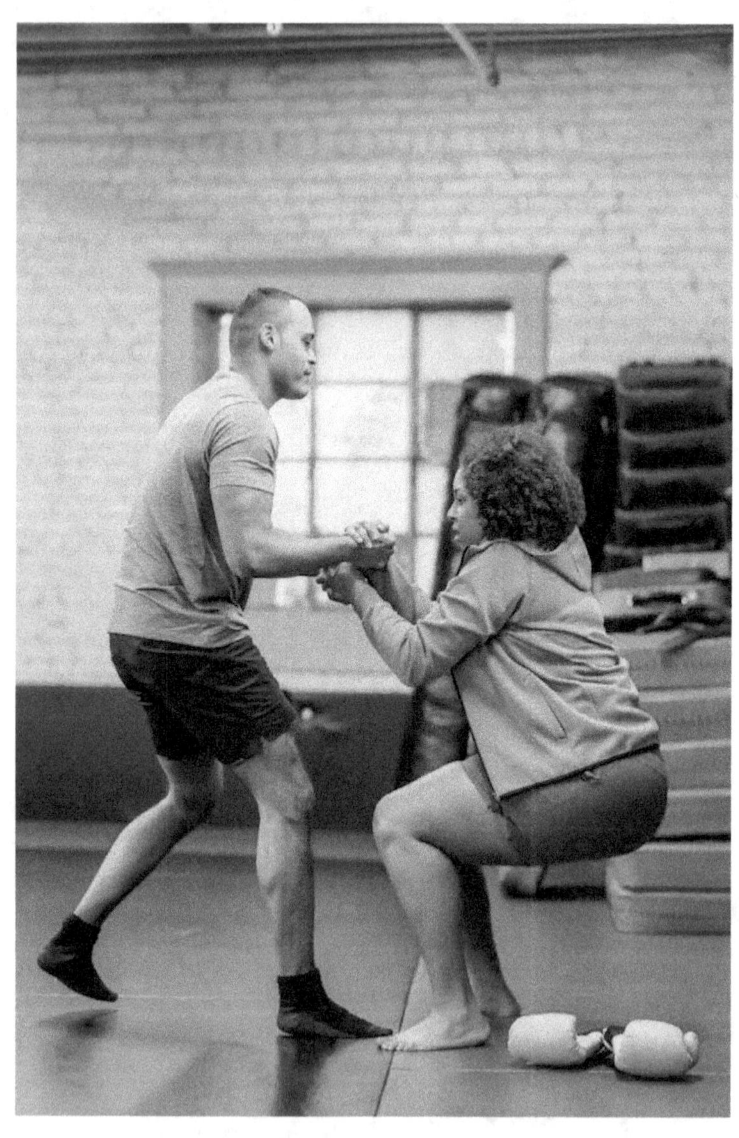

Chapter 1: Understanding Osteoporosis

Understanding Osteoporosis:

Osteoporosis is a common yet often misunderstood condition that affects the skeletal system, leading to weakened bones and increased risk of fractures. In this section, we will delve into the fundamental aspects of osteoporosis, including its definition, causes, risk factors, and impact on quality of life.

1. **Definition of Osteoporosis**: Osteoporosis is a progressive bone disease characterized by low bone mass and deterioration of bone tissue, resulting in fragile and porous bones. This condition diminishes bone strength and density, making individuals more susceptible to fractures, particularly in the spine, hips, and wrists. Osteoporosis is commonly referred to as a "silent disease" since it usually advances without any obvious signs until a fracture occurs.

2. **Causes of Osteoporosis**: The development of osteoporosis is influenced by various factors, including:

- Age: Bone density tends to decrease with age, making older adults more vulnerable to osteoporosis.
- Gender: Women, especially postmenopausal women, are at a higher risk of osteoporosis due to hormonal changes that affect bone density.
- Hormonal Changes: Decreased estrogen levels in women and testosterone levels in men can contribute to bone loss.
- Nutritional Deficiencies: A lack of calcium, vitamin D, and other critical minerals can weaken bones.
- Lifestyle Factors: Sedentary lifestyle, smoking, excessive alcohol consumption, and low body weight can negatively impact bone health.
- Medical Conditions: Certain medical conditions like thyroid disorders, gastrointestinal diseases, and hormonal imbalances can increase the risk of osteoporosis.

3. **Risk Factors for Osteoporosis:** Understanding the risk factors associated with

osteoporosis is crucial for early detection and prevention. Common risk factors include:

- Family History: Individuals with a family history of osteoporosis or fractures are more likely to develop the disorder.

- Gender and Age: Women over 50 and men over 70 are at higher risk, although osteoporosis can affect individuals of any age.
- Menopause: Women experience accelerated bone loss after menopause due to hormonal changes.
- Low Body Weight: Having a low body weight or a small frame increases the risk of osteoporosis.
- Sedentary Lifestyle: Lack of physical activity and exercise contributes to bone weakening.
- Smoking and Alcohol: Smoking tobacco and excessive alcohol consumption can impair bone health.
- Medications: Certain medications, such as corticosteroids and long-term use of proton pump inhibitors, can increase the risk of osteoporosis.

4. **Impact on Quality of Life**: Osteoporosis can have profound implications for an individual's quality of life. The risk of fractures,

especially in weight-bearing bones, can lead to pain, limited mobility, and loss of independence. Fractures, particularly hip fractures, can also increase the risk of complications and mortality, making osteoporosis a significant health concern.

By understanding the definition, causes, risk factors, and impact of osteoporosis, individuals can take proactive steps to prevent, manage, and treat this condition. Early detection through bone density testing and adopting lifestyle modifications that promote bone health are key strategies in combating osteoporosis and preserving overall well-being.

Definition and Causes:

Definition of Osteoporosis:
Osteoporosis is a chronic bone disease characterized by decreased bone density and quality, leading to an increased risk of fractures. The term "osteoporosis" translates to "porous bones," highlighting the condition's hallmark of bone tissue becoming fragile and more susceptible to fractures. These fractures commonly occur in the spine, hips, and wrists, often resulting from minor falls or even everyday activities. The primary concern with

osteoporosis is the gradual weakening of bones over time, often without noticeable symptoms until a fracture occurs. This silent progression makes early detection and proactive management crucial in minimizing the impact of osteoporosis on an individual's quality of life.

Causes of Osteoporosis:

1. **Age-Related Bone Loss**: One of the primary causes of osteoporosis is age-related bone loss. As individuals age, their bone turnover rate decreases, leading to a gradual reduction in bone density and strength. This age-related bone loss is more pronounced in postmenopausal women due to hormonal changes that accelerate bone resorption.

2. **Hormonal Changes**: Hormonal factors play a significant role in bone health. Estrogen, a hormone that helps maintain bone density, decreases significantly in women after menopause. This decline in estrogen levels accelerates bone loss, contributing to the higher prevalence of osteoporosis in postmenopausal women. Similarly, reduced testosterone levels in older men can also lead to bone loss and osteoporosis.

3. **Nutritional Deficiencies**: Inadequate intake of essential nutrients, particularly calcium and vitamin D, can weaken bones and increase the risk of osteoporosis. Calcium is crucial for bone mineralization, while vitamin D aids in calcium absorption and bone remodeling. A diet lacking in these nutrients, coupled with poor absorption or utilization, can compromise bone health.

4. **Lifestyle Factors**: Certain lifestyle habits and environmental factors can contribute to the development of osteoporosis. These include:

- Sedentary Lifestyle: Lack of weight-bearing exercise and physical activity can lead to reduced bone density and muscle strength, increasing the risk of osteoporosis.
- Smoking: Tobacco smoking has been linked to accelerated bone loss and impaired bone healing, making smokers more susceptible to osteoporosis.
- Excessive Alcohol Consumption: Chronic alcohol abuse can interfere with calcium absorption and bone metabolism, contributing to bone loss and osteoporosis.
- Low Body Weight: Being underweight or having a low body mass index (BMI) can increase the risk of osteoporosis, as there may

be less bone mass to support the body's structure.

5. **Medical Conditions and Medications**: Certain medical conditions and medications can also predispose individuals to osteoporosis. These include:

- Endocrine Disorders: Conditions such as hyperthyroidism, Cushing's syndrome, and diabetes can affect bone metabolism and increase the risk of osteoporosis.
- Gastrointestinal Disorders: Malabsorption syndromes, inflammatory bowel disease (IBD), and gastric bypass surgery can interfere with nutrient absorption, impacting bone health.
- Medications: Long-term use of corticosteroids (e.g., prednisone), anticonvulsants, proton pump inhibitors (PPIs), and certain cancer treatments can weaken bones and contribute to osteoporosis.

Understanding the multifaceted causes of osteoporosis is essential for implementing preventive measures, early detection, and effective management strategies. By addressing modifiable risk factors, promoting bone-healthy behaviors, and seeking appropriate medical guidance, individuals can mitigate the impact of osteoporosis and maintain optimal bone health throughout their lives.

Risk Factors:

Osteoporosis is influenced by a variety of risk factors that can contribute to the Understanding these risk factors is critical to early discovery, prevention, and management. Here are some key risk factors associated with osteoporosis:

1. **Age**: Advanced age is a significant risk factor for osteoporosis. As people get older, bone density naturally decreases, leading to a higher susceptibility to fractures and bone-related issues.

2. **Gender**: Women are at a higher risk of developing osteoporosis compared to men, especially after menopause. The drop in estrogen levels during menopause accelerates bone loss, making women more vulnerable to this condition.

3. **Hormonal Changes**: Hormonal imbalances can contribute to bone loss and osteoporosis. Reduced estrogen levels in women and

decreased testosterone levels in men can weaken bones and increase fracture risk.

4. **Family History**: A family history of osteoporosis or a history of fractures can indicate a genetic predisposition to the condition. Individuals with close relatives who have osteoporosis are more likely to develop it themselves.

5. **Low Body Weight and BMI**: Having a low body weight or a low body mass index (BMI) can increase the risk of osteoporosis. People with smaller frames may have less bone mass to begin with, making them more susceptible to bone loss.

6. **Dietary Factors**: Inadequate intake of calcium and vitamin D, essential nutrients for bone health, can contribute to osteoporosis. A diet lacking in these nutrients can weaken bones and hinder bone remodeling processes.

7. **Sedentary Lifestyle**: Lack of physical activity, especially weight-bearing exercises and strength training, can lead to bone loss and decreased bone density. Engaging in regular exercise helps maintain bone strength and overall bone health.

8. **Smoking**: Tobacco smoking has been linked to accelerated bone loss and impaired bone healing. Smokers are at a higher risk of developing osteoporosis and experiencing fractures.

9. **Excessive Alcohol Consumption**: Chronic alcohol abuse can interfere with calcium absorption and bone metabolism, contributing to bone loss and osteoporosis.

10. **Certain Medical Conditions**: Certain medical conditions and treatments can increase the risk of osteoporosis. These include endocrine disorders (e.g., hyperthyroidism, Cushing's syndrome), gastrointestinal disorders (e.g., malabsorption syndromes, inflammatory bowel disease), and long-term use of medications such as corticosteroids, anticonvulsants, and proton pump inhibitors (PPIs).

11. **Previous Fractures**: Individuals who have previously experienced fractures, especially fragility fractures, are at an increased risk of future fractures and osteoporosis.

12. **Race and Ethnicity**: While osteoporosis can affect individuals of any race or ethnicity, studies have shown that Caucasians and Asians, particularly postmenopausal women of Asian descent, have a higher prevalence of osteoporosis and fractures.

By recognizing these risk factors and addressing modifiable factors such as nutrition, exercise, and lifestyle habits, individuals can take proactive steps to reduce their risk of osteoporosis and maintain optimal bone health. Regular bone density screenings, especially for those at higher risk, can also aid in early detection and intervention.

Impact on Quality of Life:

Osteoporosis, a condition characterized by weakened bones and increased susceptibility to fractures, can have a significant impact on an individual's quality of life. This impact extends beyond physical discomfort to encompass emotional, social, and psychological aspects. Here are key ways in which osteoporosis can affect quality of life:

1. **Increased Risk of Fractures**: One of the most immediate impacts of osteoporosis is the

heightened risk of fractures, particularly in weight-bearing bones such as the spine, hips, and wrists. These fractures can result from minor falls or even daily activities, leading to pain, limited mobility, and loss of independence.

2. **Chronic Pain**: Fractures associated with osteoporosis often cause chronic pain, which can be debilitating and affect daily activities. Persistent pain, especially in the spine, can also contribute to decreased quality of life and emotional distress.

3. **Decreased Mobility and Function**: Fractures and bone weakness can lead to decreased mobility and functional limitations. Activities such as walking, climbing stairs, and lifting objects may become challenging, impacting independence and overall well-being.

4. **Loss of Independence**: Osteoporosis-related fractures and mobility issues can result in a loss of independence, as individuals may require assistance with daily tasks and activities they once performed independently. This loss of autonomy can lead

to feelings of frustration, helplessness, and decreased self-esteem.

5. **Impact on Mental Health**: Living with osteoporosis can take a toll on mental health, leading to anxiety, depression, and emotional distress. Chronic pain, fear of falling, and concerns about future fractures can contribute to psychological symptoms and affect overall mental well-being.

6. **Social Isolation**: Osteoporosis-related fractures and mobility limitations may lead to social isolation. Individuals may withdraw from social activities, hobbies, and gatherings due to fear of falling or discomfort, leading to feelings of loneliness and isolation.

7. **Financial Burden**: Managing osteoporosis, including medical treatments, rehabilitation, assistive devices, and home modifications, can impose a financial burden on individuals and their families. The cost of healthcare services and related expenses can add stress and strain to quality of life.

8. **Fear of Future Fractures**: The fear of experiencing additional fractures and complications can be emotionally taxing for

individuals with osteoporosis. This fear may lead to avoidance of activities, reduced physical activity, and heightened anxiety about the future.

9. **Impact on Relationships**: Osteoporosis can affect relationships with family members, caregivers, and healthcare providers. Caregivers may experience increased stress and burden, while family dynamics may shift to accommodate the needs of the individual with osteoporosis.

10. **Reduced Quality of Sleep**: Chronic pain, discomfort, and anxiety related to osteoporosis can interfere with sleep quality and duration. Poor sleep can further exacerbate physical and emotional symptoms, affecting overall quality of life.

11. **Negative Body Image**: Changes in posture, height loss, and visible signs of osteoporosis (e.g., dowager's hump) can impact body image and self-confidence. Individuals may be self-conscious about their appearance and battle with body image issues.

It's important to recognize the multifaceted impact of osteoporosis on quality of life and to address not only the physical aspects but also the emotional, social, and psychological aspects through comprehensive healthcare, support systems, and lifestyle modifications. Rehabilitation programs, pain management strategies, emotional support, and education about osteoporosis management can all contribute to improving quality of life for individuals living with this condition.

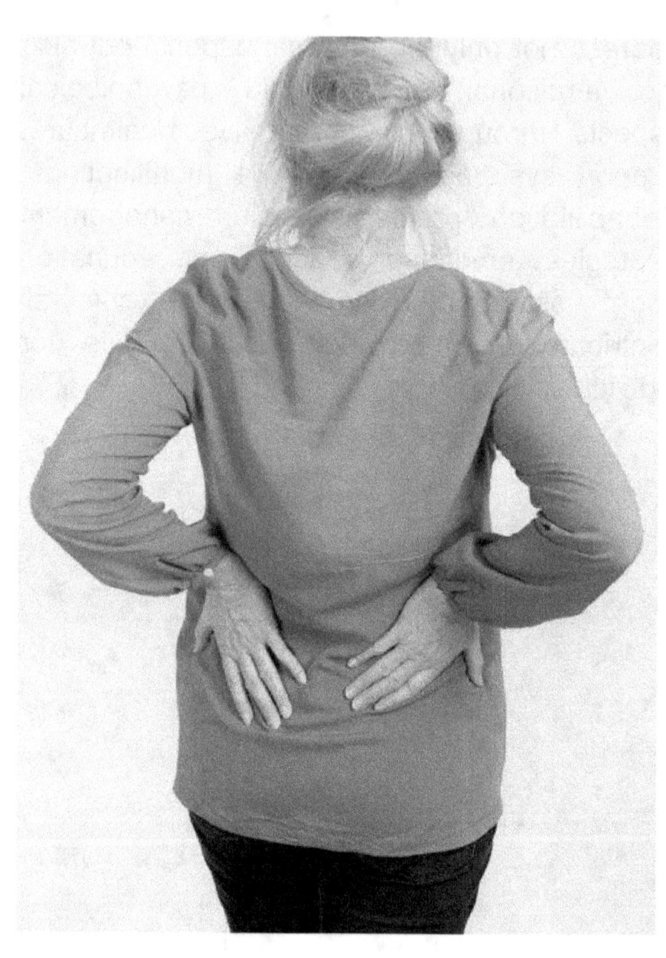

Chapter 2: Diagnosis and Assessment

Diagnosing osteoporosis involves a series of assessments and tests aimed at evaluating bone health, density, and fracture risk. Early detection is key to preventing fractures and managing osteoporosis effectively. Here are the primary methods used for diagnosis and assessment:

1. **Medical History and Physical Examination**:
   - Healthcare providers start by gathering a detailed medical history, including risk factors such as family history of osteoporosis, prior fractures, menopausal status (in women), medication use, and lifestyle factors.
   - A thorough physical examination may be conducted to assess posture, height changes, and signs of fractures or bone deformities.

2. **Bone Density Testing (Dual-Energy X-ray Absorptiometry - DXA):**
   - DXA is the gold standard for diagnosing osteoporosis and measuring bone mineral density (BMD). It is a non-invasive and painless procedure that uses low-dose X-rays

to assess bone density, typically focusing on the hip and spine.

- DXA results are reported as T-scores and Z-scores. T-scores compare an individual's BMD to that of a healthy young adult, while Z-scores compare BMD to age-matched peers.

3. **FRAX Assessment**:

- The Fracture Risk Assessment Tool (FRAX) is a widely used tool that calculates an individual's 10-year probability of major osteoporotic fractures (hip, spine, wrist, or shoulder) and hip fractures according to clinical risk factors and BMD measures.

- FRAX takes into account factors such as age, gender, BMI, previous fractures, family history, smoking status, alcohol consumption, glucocorticoid use, and secondary causes of osteoporosis.

4. **Laboratory Tests**:

- Blood tests may be conducted to assess calcium, vitamin D, parathyroid hormone (PTH), thyroid function, and other markers of bone metabolism.

- Bone turnover markers (e.g., serum CTX, serum PINP) may be measured to evaluate bone resorption and formation rates, providing additional insights into bone health.

5. **Vertebral Fracture Assessment (VFA)**:

- VFA is a specialized imaging technique that uses DXA equipment to detect vertebral fractures, particularly asymptomatic fractures in the spine. It helps identify individuals at higher risk of fractures and guides treatment decisions.

6. **Quantitative Ultrasound (QUS)**:

- QUS is an alternative method for assessing bone density and fracture risk, particularly at peripheral skeletal sites such as the heel (calcaneus). It uses sound waves to measure bone characteristics and is often used in conjunction with DXA for screening purposes.

7. **Additional Imaging Studies**:

- In some cases, additional imaging studies such as CT scans or MRI may be recommended to evaluate bone health, assess fractures, or investigate underlying conditions contributing to bone loss.

Once osteoporosis is diagnosed based on DXA results (T-score $\leq$ -2.5) or fracture risk assessments (FRAX), healthcare providers develop individualized treatment plans focused on fracture prevention, lifestyle modifications, nutritional interventions, exercise programs, and medication management. Regular monitoring and follow-up assessments are essential to track progress, adjust treatment strategies, and optimize bone health over time.

Bone Density Testing:

Bone density testing, also known as bone densitometry or Dual-Energy X-ray Absorptiometry (DXA), is a crucial component of diagnosing and assessing osteoporosis. This non-invasive and painless test measures bone mineral density (BMD) to evaluate bone health, identify osteoporosis, and assess fracture risk. Here's an overview of bone density testing in the context of osteoporosis diagnosis and assessment:

1. **Purpose of Bone Density Testing**:
   - Bone density testing is primarily used to diagnose osteoporosis, determine fracture risk, and monitor changes in bone health over time.
   - It helps healthcare providers evaluate the strength, density, and quality of bones, particularly in weight-bearing areas such as the hip and spine.

2. **Procedure**:
   - During a bone density test, the individual lies comfortably on a padded table while a specialized DXA machine emits low-dose X-rays.
   - The X-rays pass through the bones, and the amount of radiation absorbed by the bones is measured. This measurement provides information about bone density.
   - The test is quick, typically lasting 10 to 30 minutes, and does not require any special preparation or recovery time.

3. **Areas of Measurement**:
   - Bone density testing focuses on key skeletal sites, including the lumbar spine (lower back), hip (specifically the femoral neck and total hip), and sometimes the forearm (radius).
   - These areas are chosen because they are prone to fractures in individuals with osteoporosis, making them important indicators of bone health and fracture risk.

4. **Interpretation of Results**:
   - Bone density test results are reported as T-scores and Z-scores. T-scores compare an individual's BMD to that of a healthy young adult of the same gender, while Z-scores compare BMD to age-matched peers.

- A T-score of -1.0 or above is considered normal, between -1.0 and -2.5 indicates low bone density (osteopenia), and -2.5 or lower indicates osteoporosis.

- Z-scores, on the other hand, compare BMD to age-matched peers and provide insights into bone health relative to the individual's age group and demographics.

5. **Clinical Application**:

- Bone density testing plays a crucial role in guiding osteoporosis management and treatment decisions. Individuals with low bone density or osteoporosis may require lifestyle modifications, nutritional interventions, exercise programs, and medication therapy to prevent fractures and improve bone health.

- Regular follow-up bone density tests are recommended to monitor treatment efficacy, track changes in bone density, and adjust management strategies as needed.

6. **Limitations and Considerations**:

- While bone density testing is a valuable tool in osteoporosis diagnosis and assessment, it has limitations. It does not provide information about bone structure, quality, or the presence of non-osteoporotic fractures.

- Healthcare providers consider other factors such as clinical risk factors, fracture history, lifestyle habits, and overall health when evaluating fracture risk and developing comprehensive treatment plans.

Bone density testing, alongside clinical assessments and fracture risk evaluations, plays a vital role in identifying osteoporosis, guiding treatment decisions, and promoting bone health in individuals at risk for fractures and bone-related complications.

Fracture Risk Assessment

Fracture risk assessment is a crucial component of diagnosing and evaluating osteoporosis. It involves evaluating an individual's risk of experiencing fractures, particularly major osteoporotic fractures (hip, spine, wrist, or shoulder fractures) and hip fractures, over a specified period. Fracture risk assessment tools, such as the Fracture Risk Assessment Tool (FRAX), aid healthcare providers in identifying individuals at higher risk and guiding treatment decisions. Here's an in-depth look at fracture risk assessment in the context of osteoporosis diagnosis and assessment:

1. **Purpose of Fracture Risk Assessment**:
   - Fracture risk assessment aims to estimate an individual's likelihood of experiencing fractures, particularly fragility fractures associated with osteoporosis, within a specified timeframe (usually 10 years).
   - The assessment helps healthcare providers identify high-risk individuals who may benefit from interventions to prevent fractures, such as lifestyle modifications, pharmacological treatments, and fall prevention strategies.

2. **Fracture Risk Assessment Tools**:
   - The Fracture Risk Assessment Tool (FRAX) is one of the most widely used tools for evaluating fracture risk in osteoporosis. FRAX calculates an individual's 10-year probability of major osteoporotic fractures and hip fractures based on clinical risk factors and, in some cases, bone mineral density (BMD) measurements.
   - FRAX takes into account factors such as age, gender, BMI, previous fractures, family history of fractures, smoking status, alcohol consumption, glucocorticoid use, and secondary causes of osteoporosis (e.g., rheumatoid arthritis, diabetes).

3. **Clinical Risk Factors Considered in FRAX**:

- Age: Older age is a significant risk factor for osteoporosis and fractures.

- Gender: Women, especially postmenopausal women, have a higher fracture risk.

- BMI: Low body mass index (BMI) is associated with increased fracture risk.

- Previous Fractures: A history of fragility fractures increases the likelihood of future fractures.

- Family History: Having a family history of fractures, particularly in first-degree relatives, is a risk factor.

- Smoking: Tobacco smoking is linked to bone loss and higher fracture risk.

- Alcohol Consumption: Excessive alcohol intake can weaken bones and increase fracture risk.

- Glucocorticoid Use: Long-term use of corticosteroids is a known risk factor for osteoporosis and fractures.

- Secondary Causes: Certain medical conditions and medications can contribute to bone loss and fracture risk.

4. **Interpretation of FRAX Results**:

- FRAX calculates an individual's 10-year probability of major osteoporotic fractures and hip fractures as percentages.
- Healthcare providers use FRAX results, along with clinical judgment and other assessment tools (such as bone density testing), to determine fracture risk categories (low, moderate, high) and guide treatment decisions.
- Treatment thresholds for pharmacological interventions are often based on FRAX results, with higher-risk individuals recommended for osteoporosis medications to reduce fracture risk.

5. **Integration with Bone Density Testing**:
- FRAX can be used independently or in conjunction with bone density testing (DXA) to assess fracture risk more accurately.
- In cases where BMD measurements are available, FRAX with BMD incorporates bone density data into the fracture risk assessment, providing a more comprehensive evaluation of fracture risk.

6. **Clinical Application and Treatment Decisions**:
- Fracture risk assessment, including the use of FRAX, plays a crucial role in guiding

osteoporosis management and treatment decisions.

- Individuals identified as high risk for fractures may benefit from interventions such as lifestyle modifications (e.g., exercise, nutrition), fall prevention strategies, pharmacological treatments (e.g., bisphosphonates, denosumab), and regular monitoring of bone health.

- Treatment decisions are individualized based on fracture risk, overall health status, preferences, and potential benefits and risks of interventions.

Fracture risk assessment, particularly with tools like FRAX, enhances the precision of osteoporosis diagnosis and enables healthcare providers to tailor interventions that reduce fracture risk and improve bone health in at-risk individuals. Regular monitoring and reassessment of fracture risk are essential components of comprehensive osteoporosis care.

Laboratory Tests for Bone Health:

Laboratory tests play a crucial role in assessing bone health and evaluating factors that may contribute to osteoporosis. These tests provide valuable insights into bone metabolism, mineralization, and overall bone health status. Here's an overview of the laboratory tests commonly used in the diagnosis and assessment of osteoporosis:

1. Calcium and Phosphate Levels:

- Serum calcium and phosphate levels are measured to evaluate mineralization and homeostasis in bones. Abnormalities in these levels can indicate underlying metabolic bone disorders or conditions affecting calcium absorption and utilization.

2. Vitamin D Levels:

- Serum 25-hydroxyvitamin D (25(OH)D) levels are assessed to determine vitamin D status, which is crucial for calcium absorption, bone mineralization, and overall bone health. Low vitamin D levels are associated with increased fracture risk and impaired bone metabolism.

3. **Parathyroid Hormone (PTH)**:

- PTH levels are measured to assess parathyroid gland function and calcium regulation. Elevated PTH levels may indicate hyperparathyroidism, a condition that can lead to bone loss and osteoporosis.

4. **Thyroid Function Tests**:

- Thyroid function tests, including thyroid-stimulating hormone (TSH), free thyroxine (T4), and triiodothyronine (T3) levels, help evaluate thyroid gland function. Thyroid disorders such as hyperthyroidism and hypothyroidism can impact bone metabolism and contribute to bone loss.

5. **Bone Turnover Markers**:

- Bone turnover markers (BTMs) are biochemical markers that reflect the rate of bone formation and resorption. Common BTMs include serum C-terminal telopeptide of type I collagen (CTX) and serum N-terminal propeptide of type I collagen (PINP).

- Elevated levels of BTMs indicate increased bone turnover, which may occur in conditions such as osteoporosis, hyperparathyroidism, and Paget's disease. Monitoring BTMs can provide insights into bone remodeling processes and response to treatment.

6. **Renal Function Tests**:

   - Kidney function tests, including serum creatinine, blood urea nitrogen (BUN), and estimated glomerular filtration rate (eGFR), are important in assessing renal function. Chronic kidney disease (CKD) can impact mineral metabolism, leading to bone disorders and increased fracture risk.

7. **Other Metabolic Markers**:

   - Additional metabolic markers may be evaluated, including serum alkaline phosphatase (ALP), serum albumin, and serum electrolytes (e.g., potassium, magnesium). These markers help assess overall metabolic status and potential contributors to bone health.

8. **Dual-Energy X-ray Absorptiometry (DXA) Results**:

   - While not a laboratory test per se, DXA results (bone density measurements) are often integrated with laboratory findings to comprehensively evaluate bone health and fracture risk. DXA results provide information about bone mineral density (BMD) and help classify individuals as normal, osteopenic, or osteoporotic based on T-scores.

Interpreting laboratory test results in conjunction with clinical assessments, imaging studies (e.g., DXA), and fracture risk assessment tools (e.g., FRAX) enables healthcare providers to evaluate bone health comprehensively, identify underlying conditions contributing to bone loss, and tailor treatment strategies for individuals at risk for osteoporosis and fractures. Regular monitoring of laboratory parameters is essential in managing osteoporosis and optimizing bone health outcomes.

Part I: Dietary Strategies

Diet is essential for preserving bone health and preventing osteoporosis. Adequate intake of essential nutrients, particularly calcium, vitamin D, magnesium, and vitamin K, is vital for optimal bone mineralization, strength, and density. Here's an overview of dietary strategies used in the diagnosis and assessment of osteoporosis:

1. **Calcium Intake**:
   - Calcium is a key mineral essential for bone formation and strength. Adequate calcium intake throughout life is important for building and maintaining healthy bones.
   - Recommended daily calcium intake varies by age and gender but generally ranges from 1,000 to 1,200 milligrams (mg) for most adults. Postmenopausal women and older adults may require higher calcium intake.
   - Good dietary sources of calcium include dairy products (e.g., milk, yogurt, cheese), leafy green vegetables (e.g., kale, broccoli), fortified foods (e.g., fortified cereals, orange juice), and calcium-rich seafood (e.g., canned salmon with bones).

2. **Vitamin D Supplementation**:
   - Vitamin D plays a crucial role in calcium absorption and bone mineralization. Adequate vitamin D levels are essential for maintaining bone health.
   - Sun exposure, fortified foods (e.g., fortified milk, cereal), and dietary supplements are sources of vitamin D. However, many individuals may require supplemental vitamin D, especially those with limited sun exposure or inadequate dietary intake.

- The recommended daily intake of vitamin D varies but typically ranges from 600 to 800 International Units (IU) for adults, with higher doses recommended for certain populations, such as older adults and individuals with vitamin D deficiency.

3. Magnesium and Vitamin K:

- Magnesium is involved in bone mineralization and plays a role in calcium metabolism. Consuming magnesium-rich foods such as nuts, seeds, whole grains, and leafy greens supports bone health.

- Vitamin K is essential for bone formation and helps activate proteins involved in bone mineralization. Good dietary sources of vitamin K include leafy green vegetables (e.g., spinach, kale), broccoli, Brussels sprouts, and fermented foods (e.g., natto).

- Including magnesium and vitamin K-rich foods in the diet contributes to overall bone health and may support bone density.

4. Protein and Micronutrients:

- Adequate protein intake is important for maintaining muscle mass and supporting bone health. Incorporating lean sources of protein such as poultry, fish, legumes, and tofu can benefit bone health.

- Other micronutrients, such as phosphorus, potassium, zinc, and vitamin C, also play roles in bone metabolism and overall health. Consuming a varied and balanced diet that includes a variety of fruits, vegetables, whole grains, and lean proteins provides essential nutrients for bone health.

5. **Limiting Sodium and Caffeine**:

- High sodium intake can lead to calcium excretion and may contribute to bone loss. Limiting processed foods, salty snacks, and excessive salt use can help reduce sodium intake.

- Excessive caffeine consumption may also affect calcium absorption and contribute to bone loss. Moderating caffeine intake from sources such as coffee, tea, and energy drinks is recommended for individuals concerned about bone health.

6. **Alcohol Moderation and Tobacco Cessation**:

- Excessive alcohol consumption can interfere with calcium absorption and bone metabolism, contributing to bone loss. Moderating alcohol intake and following recommended guidelines for alcohol consumption support bone health.

- Tobacco smoking is associated with increased bone loss and fracture risk. Quitting smoking reduces these risks and benefits overall bone health.

7. **Dietary Supplements**:

- In some cases, dietary supplements may be recommended to fill nutrient gaps or address deficiencies. Consultation with a healthcare provider or registered dietitian is recommended before starting any dietary supplements to ensure safety and effectiveness.

8. **Individualized Nutrition Plans**:

- Nutrition recommendations for osteoporosis are often individualized based on factors such as age, gender, medical history, bone density status, and dietary preferences.

- Working with a registered dietitian or healthcare provider can help develop personalized nutrition plans that optimize bone health and support overall well-being.

By adopting a balanced and nutrient-rich diet, individuals can support bone health, minimize bone loss, and reduce the risk of osteoporosis and fractures. Incorporating dietary strategies along with other lifestyle modifications and medical interventions forms a comprehensive approach to managing osteoporosis and promoting overall bone health.

Chapter 3: Essential Nutrients for Bone Health

Essential nutrients play a crucial role in supporting bone health and minimizing the risk of osteoporosis, a condition characterized by low bone mass and increased susceptibility to fractures. Incorporating these nutrients into your diet is essential for maintaining strong and healthy bones. Here are the essential nutrients for bone health, with a specific focus on their importance for preventing and managing osteoporosis:

1. **Calcium**:
   - Calcium is a fundamental mineral required for bone formation, structure, and strength. It also plays a role in muscle function, nerve transmission, and blood clotting.
   - Adequate calcium intake is vital throughout life, with particular emphasis during childhood, adolescence, and older adulthood to support bone health and prevent bone loss.
   - Good dietary sources of calcium include dairy products (milk, yogurt, cheese), leafy green vegetables (kale, broccoli), fortified

plant-based milks (soy, almond), tofu, canned fish with bones (sardines, salmon), and calcium-fortified foods (cereals, orange juice).

2. **Vitamin D:**

- Vitamin D is essential for calcium absorption and utilization in bones. It helps maintain proper calcium and phosphorus levels in the blood, promoting bone mineralization and density.

- Sun exposure stimulates vitamin D synthesis in the skin, but dietary sources and supplements are important, especially for individuals with limited sun exposure or inadequate dietary intake.

- Good dietary sources of vitamin D include fatty fish (salmon, mackerel, tuna), egg yolks, fortified foods (milk, cereal, orange juice), and vitamin D supplements as recommended by healthcare providers.

3. **Magnesium:**

- Magnesium is involved in bone metabolism and helps convert vitamin D into its active form for calcium absorption. It also contributes to maintaining bone density and strength.

- Dietary sources of magnesium include nuts (almonds, cashews), seeds (pumpkin seeds, sunflower seeds), whole grains (brown rice, quinoa), leafy green vegetables (spinach, Swiss chard), legumes, and avocados.

4. **Vitamin K:**

- Vitamin K plays a role in bone mineralization and the synthesis of proteins involved in bone formation. It helps activate osteocalcin, a protein that binds calcium to bones.

- Good dietary sources of vitamin K include leafy green vegetables (kale, collard greens, spinach), Brussels sprouts, broccoli, cabbage, parsley, and fermented foods (natto).

5. **Protein**:

- Protein is essential for building and repairing bone tissue, as well as maintaining muscle mass and strength. Adequate protein intake supports bone health and overall skeletal integrity.

- Include lean sources of protein such as poultry, fish, lean meats, legumes, tofu, tempeh, and low-fat dairy products in your diet.

6. **Omega-3 Fatty Acids:**

- Omega-3 fatty acids have anti-inflammatory properties and may help reduce bone loss and improve bone density. Include sources of omega-3s such as fatty fish (salmon, sardines), flaxseeds, chia seeds, walnuts, and algae supplements.

7. **Phosphorus**:
 - Phosphorus works with calcium to form hydroxyapatite crystals, the mineral complex that gives bones strength and structure. It plays a crucial role in bone mineralization.
 - Dietary sources of phosphorus include dairy products, meat, poultry, fish, nuts, seeds, whole grains, and legumes.

8. **Other Micronutrients**   - Micronutrients like zinc, copper, manganese, boron, and vitamin C also contribute to bone health by supporting collagen synthesis, antioxidant protection, and bone remodeling processes.
 - Consume a diverse diet rich in fruits, vegetables, whole grains, nuts, seeds, and legumes to guarantee appropriate consumption of essential micronutrients.

Incorporating a well-balanced diet that includes these essential nutrients, along with regular physical activity, weight-bearing exercises, and healthy lifestyle habits, plays a crucial role in preventing osteoporosis, maintaining bone density, and promoting overall bone health throughout life. Consulting with a healthcare provider or registered dietitian can help tailor a nutrition plan that meets your specific bone health needs and goals.

Calcium Sources and Requirements:

Calcium is a crucial mineral essential for building and maintaining strong bones and teeth. It plays a fundamental role in various physiological processes, including muscle contraction, nerve transmission, and blood clotting. Adequate calcium intake is vital throughout life, with specific emphasis during periods of rapid growth (such as childhood and adolescence) and in older adulthood to prevent bone loss and osteoporosis. Here's an overview of calcium sources, requirements, and its importance for bone health:

1. **Calcium Requirements**:
   - The recommended daily calcium intake varies depending on age, gender, and life stage. The following are general guidelines for calcium intake:
   - Children (1-3 years): 700 mg/day
   - Children (4-8 years): 1,000 mg/day

- Adolescents (9-18 years): 1,300 mg/day
- Adults (19-50 years): 1,000 mg/day
- Women (51-70 years): 1,200 mg/day
- Men (51-70 years): 1,000 mg/day
- Adults over 70: 1,200 mg per day.

2. Calcium Sources:

- Dairy Products: Milk, yogurt, and cheese are rich sources of calcium. Choose low-fat or non-fat options to limit saturated fat and calorie intake.

- Fortified Foods: Many foods are fortified with calcium, including fortified plant-based milks (soy, almond, oat), orange juice, cereals, and tofu.

- Leafy Green Vegetables: Broccoli, kale, collard greens, bok choy, and spinach are good sources of calcium, although the bioavailability may vary.

- Canned Fish with Bones: Canned sardines and salmon (with bones) provide calcium along with omega-3 fatty acids.

- Calcium-rich nuts and seeds include almonds, sesame seeds, chia seeds, and tahini.

- Legumes: Beans, lentils, and chickpeas help with calcium intake.

- Fortified Snacks: Some snacks, such as calcium-fortified granola bars and crackers, can be additional sources of calcium.

3. **Calcium Absorption Factors**:

- Vitamin D: Adequate vitamin D levels are necessary for optimal calcium absorption. Vitamin D helps regulate calcium transport in the intestines.

- Magnesium: Magnesium plays a role in calcium metabolism and may influence calcium absorption.

- Protein: Consuming sufficient protein supports calcium absorption and utilization.

- Acidic Environment: Calcium absorption is enhanced in an acidic environment, so consuming foods containing vitamin C or acidic fruits alongside calcium-rich meals can be beneficial.

- Oxalates and Phytates: Some plant foods (e.g., spinach, Swiss chard, almonds) contain oxalates and phytates that can bind to calcium and reduce absorption. However, these foods are still valuable sources of calcium and other nutrients.

4. **Calcium Supplements**:

- In cases where dietary calcium intake is inadequate, supplements may be recommended under the guidance of a healthcare provider. Calcium supplements come in various forms (calcium carbonate, calcium citrate) and should be taken with meals for better absorption.
   - It's important not to exceed the recommended daily intake of calcium from food and supplements combined, as excessive calcium intake can lead to adverse effects such as kidney stones can interfere with the absorption of other minerals.

5. **Calcium Balance and Bone Health**:
   - Calcium balance is crucial for bone health. When dietary calcium intake is insufficient, the body may draw calcium from bones, potentially leading to bone weakening and increased fracture risk.
   - Consuming adequate calcium, along with other essential nutrients like vitamin D, magnesium, and protein, supports bone mineralization, density, and strength, reducing the risk of osteoporosis and fractures.

By including a variety of calcium-rich foods in your diet, meeting recommended calcium intake levels, and ensuring factors that enhance calcium absorption are in place, you can support optimal bone health and lower the risk of bone-related disorders including osteoporosis. Regular monitoring of calcium intake and bone health, especially in vulnerable populations, is important for maintaining lifelong skeletal strength and resilience.

Vitamin D and Sunlight Exposure:

Vitamin D is a crucial nutrient that plays a significant role in bone health, immune function, and overall well-being. One of the primary sources of vitamin D is sunlight exposure, which triggers the synthesis of vitamin D in the skin. Understanding the importance of vitamin D and sunlight exposure is key to maintaining optimal bone health and preventing conditions like osteoporosis. Here's an in-depth look at vitamin D, its benefits for bone health, and how sunlight exposure contributes to vitamin D synthesis:

1. **Importance of Vitamin D for Bone Health**:
    - Vitamin D is essential for calcium absorption and utilization in the body,

particularly in the intestines. It helps regulate calcium and phosphorus levels in the blood, supporting bone mineralization, density, and strength.

- Adequate vitamin D levels are crucial for maintaining healthy bones and preventing conditions like osteoporosis, which is characterized by low bone mass and increased fracture risk.

2. **Sources of Vitamin D:**

- Sunlight Exposure: Ultraviolet B (UVB) rays from sunlight interact with a precursor molecule in the skin, converting it into vitamin D3 (cholecalciferol). This process is the primary source of vitamin D for most people.

- Dietary Sources: While sunlight exposure is the main natural source of vitamin D, certain foods are also good dietary sources. These include fatty fish (salmon, mackerel, tuna), egg yolks, fortified foods (milk, cereal, orange juice), and vitamin D supplements.

3. **Sunlight Exposure and Vitamin D Synthesis**:

- Sunlight is necessary for the production of vitamin D in the skin.

When exposed to UVB rays, a cholesterol derivative in the skin undergoes a chemical reaction, leading to the formation of vitamin D3.

- The amount of vitamin D produced by exposure to sunlight varies depending on time of day, season, latitude, skin pigmentation, and sunscreen use.

- Generally, exposing arms, legs, or face to sunlight for about 10 to 30 minutes a few times a week during peak UVB hours (10 am to 3 pm) can help maintain adequate vitamin D levels, especially in regions with sufficient UVB radiation.

4. **Factors Affecting Sunlight Exposure and Vitamin D Synthesis**:

- Latitude and Season: UVB radiation intensity varies with latitude and season. Regions closer to the equator receive more intense UVB rays throughout the year, while UVB levels decrease at higher latitudes and during winter months.

- Time of Day: UVB radiation is most intense during midday (10 am to 3 pm), making this period optimal for vitamin D synthesis through sunlight exposure.

- Skin Pigmentation: Darker skin tones have higher melanin levels, which can reduce the skin's ability to produce vitamin D in response to sunlight. Longer exposure times may be needed for individuals with darker skin.

   - Sunscreen Use: While sunscreen is essential for protecting against harmful UV radiation and reducing the risk of skin cancer, it can also inhibit vitamin D synthesis. Applying sunscreen with a sun protection factor (SPF) of 30 or higher can block UVB rays and reduce vitamin D production. However, brief unprotected exposure before applying sunscreen can still allow for vitamin D synthesis without increasing skin cancer risk significantly.

5.   Supplementation and Alternative Sources:

   - In cases where sunlight exposure is limited (due to climate, lifestyle, indoor work, or health reasons) or dietary intake is insufficient, vitamin D supplements may be recommended. These supplements come in various forms (vitamin D2, vitamin D3) and dosages, and healthcare providers can determine the appropriate supplementation based on individual needs and vitamin D levels.

   - Consuming vitamin D-rich foods and fortified products can also contribute to vitamin D intake, but sunlight exposure remains a primary natural source.

6. **Health Benefits Beyond Bone Health**:
    - In addition to supporting bone health, vitamin D plays roles in immune function, mood regulation, cardiovascular health, and cancer prevention.
    - Adequate vitamin D levels are associated with reduced risks of infections, autoimmune diseases, depression, cardiovascular diseases, and certain types of cancers.

7. **Balancing Sunlight Exposure and Sun Protection**:
    - While sunlight is essential for vitamin D synthesis, it's crucial to balance sunlight exposure with sun protection strategies to minimize the risk of skin damage and skin cancer.
    - Opt for brief, unprotected sun exposure during midday hours to facilitate vitamin D synthesis, and then apply sunscreen or seek shade to protect the skin from excessive UV radiation.
    - Wear protective clothing, hats, and sunglasses, and use sunscreen with broad-spectrum protection (UVA and UVB) and an appropriate SPF level based on skin type and sun exposure duration.

In conclusion, vitamin D is a vital nutrient for bone health, and sunlight exposure is a primary natural source of vitamin D synthesis in the body. Balancing sunlight exposure with sun protection measures, maintaining a healthy diet rich in vitamin D, and considering supplementation when necessary are key strategies for supporting optimal bone health and overall well-being. Regular monitoring of vitamin D levels and consulting with healthcare providers can help ensure adequate vitamin D status and reduce the risk of bone-related conditions like osteoporosis.

Magnesium, Vitamin K, and Other Key Nutrients:

In addition to calcium and vitamin D, several other nutrients play crucial roles in maintaining optimal bone health and reducing the risk of osteoporosis and fractures. These nutrients include magnesium, vitamin K, phosphorus, protein, and other micronutrients. Here's an overview of their importance and dietary sources:

1. **Magnesium**:
   - Importance: Magnesium is involved in bone metabolism, bone mineralization, and maintaining bone density. It also plays a role in activating vitamin D and calcium transport.
   - Dietary Sources: Magnesium-rich foods include nuts (almonds, cashews), seeds (pumpkin seeds, sunflower seeds), whole grains (brown rice, quinoa), legumes (beans, lentils), leafy green vegetables (spinach, Swiss chard), bananas, avocados, and dark chocolate.

2. **Vitamin K**:
   - Importance: Vitamin K is essential for bone formation and mineralization. It helps activate osteocalcin, a protein involved in binding calcium to bones.
   - Types: There are two main forms of vitamin K: vitamin K1 (phylloquinone) found in leafy green vegetables, and vitamin K2 (menaquinone) found in fermented foods and animal products.
   - Dietary Sources: Good sources of vitamin K1 include kale, spinach, broccoli, Brussels sprouts, and parsley. Vitamin K2 is found in fermented foods like natto (fermented soybeans), cheese, egg yolks, and certain meats.

3. **Phosphorus**:
   - Importance: Phosphorus works with calcium to form hydroxyapatite crystals, the mineral complex that gives bones strength and structure. It plays a crucial role in bone mineralization.
   - Dietary Sources: Phosphorus-rich foods include dairy products, meat, poultry, fish, nuts, seeds, whole grains, and legumes.

4. **Protein**:
   - Importance: Protein is essential for building and repairing bone tissue, as well as maintaining muscle mass and strength. Adequate protein intake supports bone health and overall skeletal integrity.
   - Dietary Sources: Lean sources of protein include poultry, fish, lean meats, legumes, tofu, tempeh, low-fat dairy products, and plant-based protein sources like beans and lentils.

5. **Other Micronutrients**:
   - Zinc: Zinc is involved in bone formation and mineralization. Meat, seafood, legumes, nuts, seeds, and whole grains are good sources.
   - **Copper:** Copper plays a role in collagen synthesis and bone mineralization. Dietary

sources include nuts, seeds, shellfish, organ meats, whole grains, and legumes.

- Manganese: Manganese contributes to bone development and maintenance. It is found in whole grains, nuts, seeds, legumes, and leafy green vegetables.

- Vitamin C: Vitamin C supports collagen production, which is essential for bone strength. Citrus fruits, strawberries, kiwi, bell peppers, and broccoli are common sources.

6. Balancing Nutrient Intake:

- Consuming a varied and balanced diet that includes a wide range of fruits, vegetables, whole grains, lean proteins, nuts, seeds, and legumes ensures adequate intake of these key nutrients for bone health.

- It's important to note that nutrient interactions and balance are crucial. For example, excessive phosphorus intake relative to calcium intake may interfere with calcium absorption and balance, so maintaining an appropriate ratio of these minerals is important.

7. Supplementation:

- While a well-rounded diet should provide most of these essential nutrients, supplementation may be necessary for individuals with specific dietary restrictions, deficiencies, or medical conditions. Consultation with a healthcare provider or registered dietitian can help determine if supplementation is needed and ensure appropriate dosages.

Incorporating these key nutrients into your diet, along with regular physical activity, weight-bearing exercises, and sun exposure for vitamin D synthesis, forms a comprehensive approach to supporting optimal bone health and reducing the risk of bone-related conditions like osteoporosis. Individualized nutrition plans and regular monitoring of bone health markers can further optimize bone health outcomes.

Chapter 4: Foods to Include and Avoid

A well-balanced diet plays a crucial role in managing osteoporosis and promoting bone health. Including nutrient-rich foods that support bone mineralization and avoiding those that may contribute to bone loss can help maintain strong and healthy bones. Here are foods to include and avoid for individuals with osteoporosis:

Foods to Include:

1. **Calcium-Rich Foods**:
   - Dairy Products: Low-fat or non-fat milk, yogurt, and cheese are excellent sources of calcium.
   - Fortified Foods: Include calcium-fortified foods such as fortified plant-based milks (soy, almond, oat), orange juice, cereals, and tofu.
   - Leafy Green Vegetables: Consume plenty of leafy greens like kale, spinach, collard greens, and broccoli for their calcium content.
   - Canned Fish with Bones: Incorporate canned sardines and salmon (with bones) into your diet for both calcium and omega-3 fatty acids.

2. **Vitamin D Sources**:

   - Fatty Fish: Include salmon, mackerel, tuna, and sardines in your diet for vitamin D and omega-3s.

   - Egg yolks include a natural source of vitamin D.

   - Fortified Foods: Consume fortified milk, cereal, orange juice, and other fortified products to boost your vitamin D intake.

3. **Magnesium-Rich Foods**:

   - Nuts and Seeds: Almonds, cashews, sunflower seeds, and pumpkin seeds are good sources of magnesium.

   - Whole Grains: Incorporate whole grains like brown rice, quinoa, whole wheat bread, and oats into your meals.

4. **Vitamin K Sources**:

   - Leafy Greens: Kale, spinach, Swiss chard, and collard greens are rich in vitamin K1.

   - Fermented Foods: Include fermented foods like natto, cheese, and certain yogurts for vitamin K2.

5. **Protein Sources**:

   - Lean Meats: Opt for lean cuts of poultry (chicken, turkey) and lean beef.

- Fish: Choose fish like salmon, trout, and tuna for protein and omega-3 fatty acids.
- Legumes: Include beans, lentils, chickpeas, and tofu for plant-based protein.

6. **Phosphorus-Rich Foods**:
- Dairy: Dairy products also provide phosphorus along with calcium.
- Meats: Lean meats, poultry, and fish are sources of phosphorus.

7. **Other Nutrient-Rich Foods**:
- Fruits and Vegetables: Consume a variety of fruits and vegetables for vitamins, minerals, and antioxidants.
- Healthy Fats: Include sources of healthy fats like avocados, olive oil, nuts, and seeds.

Foods to Avoid or Limit:

1. High-Sodium Foods:
- Processed Foods: Avoid highly processed foods like canned soups, frozen meals, and snacks with high sodium content.
- Salty Snacks: Limit intake of salty snacks such as chips, pretzels, and salted nuts.

2. Excessive Caffeine:

- Coffee and Tea: Moderate your intake of caffeinated beverages like coffee and tea, as excessive caffeine can interfere with calcium absorption.

3. Alcohol:
- Limit alcohol consumption, as excessive alcohol intake can lead to bone loss and increase fracture risk.

4. Sugary Foods and Beverages:
- Limit sugary foods and beverages like sodas, candies, desserts, and sugary snacks, as they can contribute to inflammation and may affect bone health indirectly.

5. High-Phosphorus Foods:
- While phosphorus is essential, excessive intake relative to calcium can disrupt calcium balance. Limit consumption of phosphorus-rich foods like processed meats, carbonated drinks, and some packaged foods.

6. Smoking and Tobacco:
- Avoid smoking and tobacco use, as they can weaken bones and increase the risk of fractures.

7. Excessive Vitamin A:

- High doses of vitamin A supplements may interfere with bone health. Consult with a healthcare provider before taking vitamin A supplements.

By focusing on a balanced diet rich in calcium, vitamin D, magnesium, vitamin K, protein, and other essential nutrients while minimizing intake of sodium, caffeine, alcohol, and other potential bone-depleting factors, individuals with osteoporosis can support bone health, reduce fracture risk, and enhance overall well-being. It's important to consult with a healthcare provider or registered dietitian for personalized dietary recommendations and guidance.

Bone-Friendly Foods:

Eating a diet rich in bone-friendly foods is crucial for managing osteoporosis, a condition characterized by weak and brittle bones. These foods provide essential nutrients like calcium, vitamin D, magnesium, vitamin K, protein, and other micronutrients that support bone health, mineralization, and density. Here's a comprehensive list of bone-friendly foods to include in your diet:

1. **Dairy Products**:
   - Low-fat or non-fat milk
   - Yogurt (plain, Greek, low-fat)
   - Cheese (low-fat varieties like mozzarella, cottage cheese)

2. **Fortified Foods**:
   - Calcium-fortified plant-based milks (soy, almond, oat)
   - Fortified orange juice
   - Fortified cereals

3. **Leafy Green Vegetables**:
   - Kale
   - Spinach
   - Collard greens
   - Swiss chard
   - Broccoli

4. **Canned Fish with Bones:**
   - Sardines (packed in oil or water with bones)
   - Salmon (canned with bones)

5. **Fatty Fish**:
   - Salmon
   - Mackerel
   - Tuna
   - Trout

- Sardines (fresh)

6. **Egg Yolks**:
    - Eggs (include the yolk for vitamin D)

7. **Nuts and Seeds**:
    - Almonds
    - Cashews
    - Sunflower seeds
    - Pumpkin seeds

8. **Whole Grains**:
    - Brown rice
    - Quinoa
    - Whole wheat bread
    - Oats

9. **Legumes**:
    - Beans (kidney beans, black beans, chickpeas)
    - Lentils
    - Tofu
    - Tempeh

10. **Lean Meats**:
    - Chicken breast
    - Turkey breast
    - Lean beef
    - Pork tenderloin

11. **Healthy Fats**:
   - Avocados
   - Olive oil
   - Nuts (in moderation)
   - Seeds (chia seeds, flaxseeds)

12. **Leafy Greens (Vitamin K):**
   - Kale
   - Spinach
   - Collard greens
   - Brussels sprouts

13. **Fruits and Vegetables (Vitamin C and Antioxidants):**
   - Citrus fruits (oranges, lemons, grapefruits)
   - Berries (strawberries, blueberries, raspberries)
   - Bell peppers
   - Tomatoes
   - Kiwi
   - Papaya

14. **Dried Fruits**:
   - Dried figs
   - Dried apricots
   - Dates
   - Prunes

15. **Herbs and Spices**:
   - Turmeric (anti-inflammatory properties)
   - Ginger (anti-inflammatory properties)
   - Cinnamon
   - Basil
   - Oregano
   - Thyme
   - Rosemary

16. **Seaweed and Sea Vegetables**:
   - Nori
   - Wakame
   - Kelp

17. **Dairy Alternatives (fortified)**:
   - Soy milk is supplemented with calcium and vitamin D.
   - Almond milk (fortified with calcium and vitamin D)
   - Oat milk is supplemented with calcium and vitamin D.

18. **Bone Broth:**
   - Homemade bone broth made from chicken, beef, or fish bones

These bone-friendly foods provide a range of essential nutrients that are vital for bone health, including calcium, vitamin D, magnesium, vitamin K, protein, phosphorus, zinc, copper, manganese, and vitamin C. Including a variety of these foods in your daily meals can help support bone mineralization, density, and strength, reducing the risk of fractures and improving overall bone health. It's essential to maintain a balanced and nutritious diet, along with regular physical activity, for optimal bone health management. Consulting with a healthcare provider or registered dietitian for personalized dietary recommendations is recommended, especially for individuals with osteoporosis or other bone-related conditions.

Foods That Weaken Bones:

While certain foods are beneficial for bone health, others can weaken bones and contribute to conditions like osteoporosis. These foods may lead to calcium loss, interfere with nutrient absorption, or promote inflammation, all of which can negatively impact bone density and strength. Here are some foods that weaken bones and should be limited or avoided for individuals with osteoporosis:

1. **High-Sodium Foods**:
   - Processed Foods: Foods like frozen meals, canned soups, and processed snacks often contain high levels of sodium, which can lead to calcium excretion and bone loss.
   - Salty Snacks: Chips, pretzels, and salted nuts are high in sodium and can contribute to calcium depletion.

2. **Excessive Caffeine**:
   - Coffee and Tea: Consuming too much caffeine can interfere with calcium absorption and increase calcium excretion through urine. Limiting coffee, tea, and caffeinated beverages is advisable.

3. **Alcohol**:
   - Excessive alcohol consumption can interfere with bone remodeling and lead to decreased bone density. Limit your alcohol intake and avoid binge drinking.

4. **Sugary Foods and Beverages**:
   - Sugary snacks, desserts, sodas, and sweetened beverages can contribute to inflammation and may affect calcium balance and bone health negatively. Limiting intake of these sugary foods is beneficial.

5. **High-Phosphorus Foods**:
   - While phosphorus is essential for bone health, excessive intake relative to calcium can disrupt calcium balance and lead to bone loss. Foods high in phosphorus include processed meats, carbonated drinks, and certain packaged foods.

6. **Foods High in Oxalates**:
   - Oxalates can bind to calcium in the digestive tract, reducing calcium absorption. Foods high in oxalates include spinach, rhubarb, beet greens, and certain nuts and seeds. While these foods offer other health benefits, they should be consumed in moderation, especially for individuals at risk of calcium deficiency.

7. **Excessive Vitamin A:**
   - High doses of vitamin A supplements may interfere with bone health and contribute to bone loss. It's important to consult with a healthcare provider before taking vitamin A supplements, especially if you are already at risk of osteoporosis.

8. **Acidic Foods**:
   - Some highly acidic foods, such as citrus fruits and tomatoes, can promote acidosis in

the body. While these foods are nutritious, consuming them in excess may affect calcium balance and bone health. Balance acidic foods with alkaline foods like leafy greens, vegetables, and fruits.

9. **High-Protein Diets:**

   - While protein is essential for bone health, excessive consumption of animal protein, especially red meat, may lead to increased calcium excretion and bone resorption. Aim for a balanced diet with moderate protein intake from various sources, including lean meats, fish, legumes, and plant-based proteins.

10. **Trans Fats and Saturated Fats**:

   - Foods high in trans fats and saturated fats, such as fried foods, processed meats, and full-fat dairy products, can contribute to inflammation and negatively impact bone health. Choose healthier fats like monounsaturated and polyunsaturated fats found in nuts, seeds, avocados, and olive oil.

By limiting or avoiding these bone-weakening foods and focusing on a balanced diet rich in bone-friendly nutrients like calcium, vitamin D, magnesium, vitamin K, and protein, individuals with osteoporosis can better manage their condition and support overall bone health. Consulting with a healthcare provider or registered dietitian for personalized dietary guidance is recommended, especially for those with specific dietary needs or medical conditions related to bone health.

Importance of a Balanced Diet:

A balanced diet plays a critical role in managing osteoporosis, a condition characterized by weakened and brittle bones. Osteoporosis increases the risk of fractures and can significantly impact an individual's quality of life. Adopting a balanced diet rich in essential nutrients is crucial for maintaining optimal bone health and reducing the progression of osteoporosis. Here's why a balanced diet is important for individuals with osteoporosis:

1. **Optimal Nutrient Intake**: A balanced diet provides the body with the essential nutrients needed for bone health. Key nutrients include calcium, vitamin D, magnesium, vitamin K, phosphorus, protein, and other micronutrients.

These nutrients support bone mineralization, density, and strength, reducing the risk of fractures and improving overall bone health.

2. **Calcium Absorption**: Calcium is a fundamental mineral for bone formation and structure. A balanced diet ensures adequate calcium intake and promotes optimal calcium absorption. Consuming calcium-rich foods alongside vitamin D-rich foods enhances calcium absorption, supporting bone mineralization and density.

3. **Vitamin D Synthesis**: Vitamin D is essential for calcium absorption and utilization in bones. Sunlight exposure, dietary sources, and supplements contribute to vitamin D levels. A balanced diet includes vitamin D-rich foods and promotes safe sun exposure to maintain adequate vitamin D levels, crucial for bone health.

4. **Magnesium and Vitamin K:** These nutrients play vital roles in bone metabolism, mineralization, and maintaining bone density. Including magnesium-rich foods (nuts, seeds, whole grains) and vitamin K-rich foods (leafy greens, fermented foods) supports bone health and reduces the risk of fractures.

5. **Protein for Bone Strength**: Adequate protein intake supports bone formation, repair, and maintenance. A balanced diet includes lean protein sources like poultry, fish, legumes, and tofu, promoting bone strength and integrity.

6. **Balanced pH Levels**: Acidic and alkaline foods affect the body's pH balance. Excessive consumption of acidic foods (like red meat, processed foods) can lead to acidosis, affecting calcium balance and bone health. A balanced diet includes alkaline-forming foods (fruits, vegetables) to maintain a healthy pH balance.

7. **Reducing Bone-Weakening Factors**: A balanced diet helps limit or avoid bone-weakening factors like excessive sodium, caffeine, alcohol, and sugary foods. These factors can contribute to calcium loss, interfere with nutrient absorption, and promote inflammation, negatively impacting bone density and strength.

8. **Overall Health and Well-being**: A balanced diet not only supports bone health but also promotes overall health and well-being. It provides essential nutrients for immune

function, cardiovascular health, muscle strength, and cognitive function, contributing to a healthier lifestyle.

9. **Weight Management**: Maintaining a healthy weight through a balanced diet and regular physical activity reduces the risk of osteoporosis-related fractures. Excess body weight can strain bones, while inadequate weight can lead to bone loss, highlighting the importance of a balanced diet in weight management and bone health.

10. **Individualized Nutrition Plans**: Consulting with a healthcare provider or registered dietitian helps create individualized nutrition plans tailored to specific bone health needs, dietary preferences, and lifestyle factors. Personalized nutrition guidance optimizes nutrient intake, supports bone health management, and enhances overall quality of life for individuals with osteoporosis.

In conclusion, a balanced diet is essential for managing osteoporosis and promoting optimal bone health. By including a variety of nutrient-rich foods, prioritizing bone-friendly nutrients, and minimizing bone-weakening factors, individuals with osteoporosis can support bone mineralization, reduce fracture risk, and improve overall well-being. Regular monitoring, dietary adjustments, and professional guidance ensure effective management of osteoporosis through nutrition.

Part II: Exercise and Physical Activity

Exercise and physical activity play crucial roles in managing osteoporosis, a condition characterized by weakened and brittle bones. Incorporating regular exercise into your routine can help improve bone density, strength, balance, and overall quality of life. Here's how exercise and physical activity benefit individuals with osteoporosis:

1. **Strength Training**:
   - Weight-bearing and resistance exercises are particularly beneficial for building and maintaining bone density and muscle strength.
   - Weight-bearing exercises include walking, jogging, hiking, dancing, stair climbing, and aerobics, which help stimulate bone growth and reduce bone loss.

- Resistance training using weights, resistance bands, or bodyweight exercises (like squats, lunges, push-ups) strengthens muscles and bones, reducing the risk of falls and fractures.

2. Balance and Stability Exercises:
- Balance and stability exercises improve coordination, proprioception, and posture, reducing the risk of falls and fractures.
- Examples include standing on one leg, heel-to-toe walking, Tai Chi, yoga, and Pilates, which enhance balance, flexibility, and core strength.

3. Flexibility and Range of Motion Exercises:
- Stretching exercises improve flexibility, joint mobility, and range of motion, reducing stiffness and preventing injuries.
- Include stretching routines for major muscle groups, such as shoulders, back, hips, and legs, to maintain mobility and prevent muscle imbalances.

4. Aerobic Exercise:
- Low-impact aerobic activities like swimming, cycling, elliptical training, and water

aerobics provide cardiovascular benefits without stressing the bones.

- Aerobic exercise improves heart health, lung function, circulation, and overall fitness, contributing to better overall health for individuals with osteoporosis.

5. **Functional Training**:

- Functional exercises mimic daily activities and movements, enhancing functional capacity, independence, and confidence in performing daily tasks.

- Examples include lifting groceries, bending to pick up objects, climbing stairs, and getting in and out of chairs safely.

6. **Safety Tips for Exercise**:

- Consult with a healthcare provider or physical therapist before starting an exercise program, especially if you have existing health conditions or concerns.

- Start slowly and gradually increase the intensity, duration, and frequency of your workouts to prevent injuries.

- Use proper form and technique during exercises to avoid strain or stress on joints and bones.

- Wear appropriate footwear with good support and traction to reduce the risk of falls.

- Stay hydrated and take breaks as needed during exercise sessions.

7. **Incorporating Weight-Bearing Activities**:
   - Engage in weight-bearing activities that involve impact or resistance on bones, such as walking, jogging, dancing, or using resistance equipment.
   - Aim for at least 30 minutes of moderate-intensity exercise most days of the week, or as recommended by your healthcare provider.

8. **Progressive Overload and Variety**:
   - Incorporate progressive overload by gradually increasing the intensity, duration, or resistance of your workouts to continue challenging your bones and muscles.
   - Include a variety of exercises to target different muscle groups, prevent boredom, and promote overall fitness and well-being.

9. **Posture and Body Mechanics**:
   - Focus on maintaining good posture and practicing proper body mechanics during daily activities and exercises to reduce strain on bones and joints.

- Avoid activities or movements that involve excessive bending, twisting, or heavy lifting that may increase the risk of fractures.

10. **Regular Monitoring and Adaptation**:
   - Regularly assess your progress, symptoms, and any changes in bone health with healthcare professionals.
   - Modify exercise programs as needed based on your individual needs, health status, and response to exercise.

In conclusion, exercise and physical activity are essential components of osteoporosis management, helping to improve bone density, strength, balance, and overall functional capacity. By incorporating a well-rounded exercise program that includes strength training, balance exercises, flexibility work, aerobic activities, and functional movements, individuals with osteoporosis can enhance bone health, reduce fracture risk, and improve overall quality of life. It's important to tailor exercise programs to individual needs, seek professional guidance, and prioritize safety during exercise sessions.

Chapter 5: Importance of Physical Activity

Physical activity plays a crucial role in preventing and managing osteoporosis, a condition characterized by weakened and brittle bones. Engaging in regular physical activity throughout life is essential for building and maintaining bone density, strength, and overall musculoskeletal health. Here are key reasons why physical activity is important in the fight against osteoporosis:

1. Stimulates Bone Growth: Weight-bearing and resistance exercises stimulate bone remodeling and growth, leading to increased bone density and strength. These exercises create mechanical stress on bones, prompting them to adapt and become stronger over time.

2. Reduces Bone Loss: Physical activity helps slow down the rate of bone loss that naturally occurs with age. Weight-bearing activities like walking, jogging, dancing, and weightlifting are particularly effective in preserving bone mass.

3. Improves Muscle Strength: Strong muscles provide support and protection to bones, reducing the risk of fractures. Resistance training exercises, such as lifting weights or using resistance bands, build muscle mass and strength, supporting bone health.

4. Enhances Balance and Stability: Balance and stability exercises improve coordination, proprioception, and posture, reducing the risk of falls and fractures, which are common concerns for individuals with osteoporosis.

5. Promotes Flexibility and Range of Motion: Stretching and flexibility exercises maintain joint mobility, reduce stiffness, and prevent musculoskeletal injuries. Improved flexibility also enhances overall movement and functional capacity.

6. Boosts Bone Health Across Lifespan: Engaging in physical activity from childhood through adulthood contributes to optimal bone development and peak bone mass. This foundation of strong bones built during youth can help lower the risk of osteoporosis later in life.

7. Supports Overall Health: Regular physical activity has numerous health benefits beyond bone health. It improves cardiovascular fitness, lowers blood pressure, enhances mood, reduces stress, supports weight management, and boosts immune function, contributing to overall well-being.

8. Combats Sedentary Lifestyle Effects: Sedentary behavior, such as prolonged sitting or lack of physical activity, can accelerate bone loss and weaken muscles. Regular movement and exercise counteract the negative effects of a sedentary lifestyle on bone health.

9. Customized Exercise Programs: Physical activity can be tailored to individual needs, preferences, and abilities. Healthcare professionals, such as physical therapists or exercise physiologists, can design personalized exercise programs that address specific bone health goals and limitations.

10. Lifestyle Integration: Incorporating physical activity into daily life promotes a more active lifestyle overall. Simple habits like taking the stairs instead of the elevator, walking or biking instead of driving short distances, and

participating in recreational activities or sports all contribute to better bone health.

11. Long-Term Benefits: Consistency in physical activity leads to long-term benefits for bone health. Even moderate-intensity activities performed regularly can make a significant difference in bone density, strength, and fracture prevention over time.

12. Collaboration with Healthcare Professionals: Working with healthcare providers, physical therapists, or fitness professionals ensures safe and effective exercise programming tailored to individual needs, medical history, and bone health status.

In conclusion, physical activity is a cornerstone in the prevention and management of osteoporosis. Regular exercise that includes weight-bearing activities, resistance training, balance exercises, and flexibility work supports bone health, muscle strength, and overall well-being. By making physical activity a priority throughout life and incorporating diverse forms of exercise, individuals can reduce the risk of osteoporosis-related complications and enjoy a healthier, more active lifestyle.

Weight-Bearing Exercises:

Weight-bearing exercises are crucial for individuals with osteoporosis as they help improve bone density, strength, and overall bone health. These exercises involve bearing your body weight and can be done in various forms to suit different fitness levels and preferences. Here are the benefits and examples of weight-bearing exercises for osteoporosis:

Benefits of Weight-Bearing Exercises:
1. Stimulate Bone Growth: Weight-bearing exercises create stress on bones, prompting them to adapt and become stronger. This stimulation helps stimulate bone growth and increase bone density, reducing the risk of fractures.

2. Maintain Bone Density: Regular weight-bearing activities help slow down bone loss that occurs with age and osteoporosis. Consistent exercise preserves bone density and supports overall bone health.

3. Build Muscle Strength: Weight-bearing exercises not only benefit bones but also strengthen muscles. Strong muscles provide

support and protection to bones, reducing the risk of falls and fractures.

4. Enhance Balance and Coordination: Weight-bearing activities that involve balance and coordination, such as walking or dancing, improve balance, proprioception, and overall stability, reducing the risk of falls.

5. Improve Overall Fitness: Incorporating weight-bearing exercises into your routine improves cardiovascular fitness, endurance, and overall physical fitness, contributing to a healthier lifestyle.

Examples of Weight-Bearing Exercises:

1. Walking: Walking is a simple yet effective weight-bearing exercise that can be done almost anywhere. Aim for brisk walking for at least 30 minutes most days of the week to reap bone health benefits.

2. Jogging or Running: For those capable of higher impact activities, jogging or running provides excellent bone-stimulating benefits. Start at a pace that is comfortable and gradually increase intensity as fitness improves.

3. Stair Climbing: Climbing stairs is a weight-bearing activity that engages multiple muscle groups and promotes bone strength. Use stairs instead of elevators whenever possible or incorporate stair climbing into your workout routine.

4. Dancing: Dancing is a fun and engaging way to get weight-bearing exercise. Whether it's ballroom dancing, Zumba, salsa, or hip-hop, dancing challenges balance, coordination, and bone health.

5. Jumping Rope: Jumping rope is a high-impact weight-bearing exercise that strengthens bones and improves cardiovascular fitness. Start with shorter intervals and gradually increase duration as you build stamina.

6. Hiking: Hiking on uneven terrain provides a natural form of weight-bearing exercise. It engages muscles, challenges balance, and exposes you to the benefits of outdoor activity.

7. Aerobic Classes: Participate in aerobic classes like aerobics, step aerobics, or cardio dance classes that incorporate weight-bearing

movements to enhance bone health and cardiovascular fitness.

8. Tennis or Racquet Sports: Playing tennis, racquetball, or other racquet sports involves weight-bearing movements and dynamic activities that benefit bone health and overall fitness.

9. Strength Training: Incorporate strength training exercises using body weight, resistance bands, or free weights to complement weight-bearing activities and build muscle strength.

10. Group Fitness Classes: Join group fitness classes that include weight-bearing exercises such as bodyweight exercises, lunges, squats, and leg presses to target major muscle groups and bones.

Safety Tips for Weight-Bearing Exercises:

- Start gradually and progress slowly to avoid overexertion or injury.
- Use proper footwear with good support and cushioning to reduce impact on joints.

- Maintain proper form and technique during exercises to prevent strain or stress on bones and muscles.
- Consult with a healthcare provider or physical therapist for personalized exercise recommendations, especially if you have existing health conditions or concerns.

Incorporating weight-bearing exercises into your regular routine, along with other forms of physical activity, is key to promoting bone health, reducing fracture risk, and enhancing overall well-being for individuals with osteoporosis. Tailor your exercise program to your fitness level, preferences, and safety considerations, and enjoy the benefits of a stronger, healthier body.

Resistance Training for Bone Strength:

Resistance training, also known as strength training or weightlifting, is a highly effective form of exercise for improving bone strength, density, and overall musculoskeletal health in individuals with osteoporosis. Unlike aerobic activities that primarily benefit cardiovascular fitness, resistance training specifically targets bone and muscle health, making it an essential component of osteoporosis management. Here's an overview of resistance training for bone strength and its benefits:

Benefits of Resistance Training for Bone Strength:

1. Stimulates Bone Growth: Resistance training involves applying external resistance to bones through weightlifting, resistance bands, or bodyweight exercises. This stress on bones stimulates bone remodeling, leading to increased bone density and strength.

2. Builds Muscle Mass: Resistance exercises not only strengthen bones but also build muscle mass and strength. Strong muscles provide support and protection to bones, reducing the risk of fractures and improving overall functional capacity.

3. Improves Bone Density: Consistent resistance training helps maintain or

increase bone density, reducing the rate of bone loss associated with osteoporosis and aging.

4. Enhances Balance and Coordination: Many resistance exercises involve functional movements that improve balance, coordination, and stability, reducing the risk of falls and fractures.

5. Increases Metabolic Rate: Building muscle through resistance training increases metabolic rate, which can aid in weight management and overall metabolic health.

6. Promotes Joint Health: Resistance exercises that target joint mobility and stability contribute to joint health, reducing the risk of osteoarthritis and other joint-related issues.

7. Boosts Confidence and Well-being: Improvements in strength, mobility, and overall fitness from resistance training can boost confidence, enhance mood, and improve quality of life.

Examples of Resistance Training Exercises for Bone Strength:

1. Bodyweight Exercises:
   - Squats
   - Lunges
   - Push-ups
   - Planks
   - Wall sits
   - Bodyweight rows

2. Free Weight Exercises:
   - Dumbbell squats
   - Dumbbell lunges
   - Chest presses
   - Bent-over rows
   - Shoulder presses
   - Bicep curls
   - Tricep extensions

3. Resistance Band Exercises:
   - Band squats
   - Band lunges
   - Band rows
   - Band chest presses
   - Band shoulder raises

- Band leg curls

4. Machine-Based Exercises:
   - Leg press
   - Leg extension
   - Leg curl
   - Chest press machine
   - Lat pulldown machine
   - Seated row machine
   - Shoulder press machine

5. Functional Training:

   - Functional exercises using kettlebells, medicine balls, or cable machines that mimic daily movements and improve overall functional capacity.

Safety Tips for Resistance Training:

- Begin with moderate weights or resistance and progressively increase as strength develops.
- Focus on suitable form and technique to avoid injuries and maximize benefits.
- Incorporate a variety of exercises that target different muscle groups and bone-loading patterns.

- Allow adequate rest between workouts for recovery and muscle repair.
- Listen to your body and modify exercises as needed based on comfort and ability.

Consultation with a Healthcare Professional:

Before starting a resistance training program, especially if you have osteoporosis or other medical conditions, it's important to consult with a healthcare professional, such as a physical therapist or exercise physiologist. They can assess your bone health, recommend appropriate exercises, provide guidance on proper technique, and tailor a program to your individual needs and goals.

To summarize, resistance training is an important and effective technique for improving bone strength, density, and overall musculoskeletal health in people with osteoporosis.
By incorporating a variety of resistance exercises into your fitness routine, you can enhance bone health, reduce fracture risk,

and improve overall physical function and well-being.

Flexibility and Balance Exercises:

Flexibility and balance exercises are integral components of a well-rounded exercise program for individuals with osteoporosis. These types of exercises help improve joint mobility, enhance stability, reduce the risk of falls, and support overall bone health. Here's an overview of flexibility and balance exercises for osteoporosis and their benefits:

Benefits of Flexibility and Balance Exercises:

1. Improved Joint Mobility: Flexibility exercises increase the range of motion in joints, which is beneficial for maintaining joint health and preventing stiffness or tightness.

2. Enhanced Stability and Coordination: Balance exercises challenge proprioception and coordination, improving balance and reducing the risk of falls. This is particularly

important for individuals with osteoporosis, as falls can lead to fractures.

3. Reduced Risk of Falls: By improving balance, stability, and coordination, flexibility and balance exercises help reduce the risk of falls, which is crucial for individuals with osteoporosis who may be more susceptible to fractures.

4. Enhanced Posture: Flexibility exercises that target muscles involved in posture, such as the back, shoulders, and hips, can help improve posture and reduce strain on the spine.

5. Relaxation and Stress Reduction: Many flexibility exercises incorporate breathing techniques and relaxation, promoting stress reduction and overall well-being.

Examples of Flexibility Exercises for Osteoporosis:

1. Stretching Exercises:
   - Neck stretches
   - Shoulder stretches
   - Chest stretches
   - Upper back stretches
   - Lower back stretches

- Hamstring stretches
- Quadriceps stretches
- Calf stretches
- Hip flexor stretches

2. Yoga and Pilates:
- Yoga poses (such as downward dog, warrior poses, and tree pose) improve flexibility, strength, and balance.
- Pilates exercises (such as pelvic tilts, bridges, and leg circles) focus on core strength, stability, and posture.

3. Tai Chi and Qigong:
- Tai Chi and Qigong are mind-body practices that combine slow, flowing movements with deep breathing and mindfulness. They improve balance, coordination, and relaxation.

4. Foam Rolling:
- Foam rolling is a form of self-myofascial release that helps reduce muscle tightness and improve flexibility. Focus on rolling major muscle groups gently.

Examples of Balance Exercises for Osteoporosis:

1. Single-Leg Stands:

- Stand on one leg for a few seconds, then switch to the other leg. Use a chair or a wall for support if necessary.

2. Heel-to-Toe Walks:
   - Walk in a straight line placing the heel of one foot directly in front of the toes of the other foot, like walking on a tightrope.

3. Balance Board or Balance Pad Exercises:
   - Use a balance board or balance pad to challenge stability and improve proprioception.

4. Tai Chi and Qigong Movements:
   - Tai Chi and Qigong include specific movements that challenge balance and coordination, such as weight shifts, leg lifts, and turns.

5. Stability Ball Exercises:
   - Perform exercises on a stability ball, such as seated or kneeling exercises, to improve core stability and balance.

Safety Tips for Flexibility and Balance Exercises:
- Warm up before stretching or performing balance exercises to prepare muscles and joints.

- To avoid strain or injury, use favorable form and technique while exercising.
- Start with easier variations of exercises and progress gradually as strength and balance improve.
- Use support, such as a chair or wall, when needed to maintain balance and safety.
- Listen to your body and avoid pushing beyond your comfort level to prevent falls or overexertion.

Incorporating Flexibility and Balance Exercises:

Include flexibility and balance exercises as part of your overall exercise routine for osteoporosis management. Aim for at least 2-3 days per week of flexibility exercises and balance exercises to reap the benefits for joint health, stability, and fall prevention. Consulting with a physical therapist or fitness professional can help design a customized exercise program tailored to your specific needs, abilities, and goals.

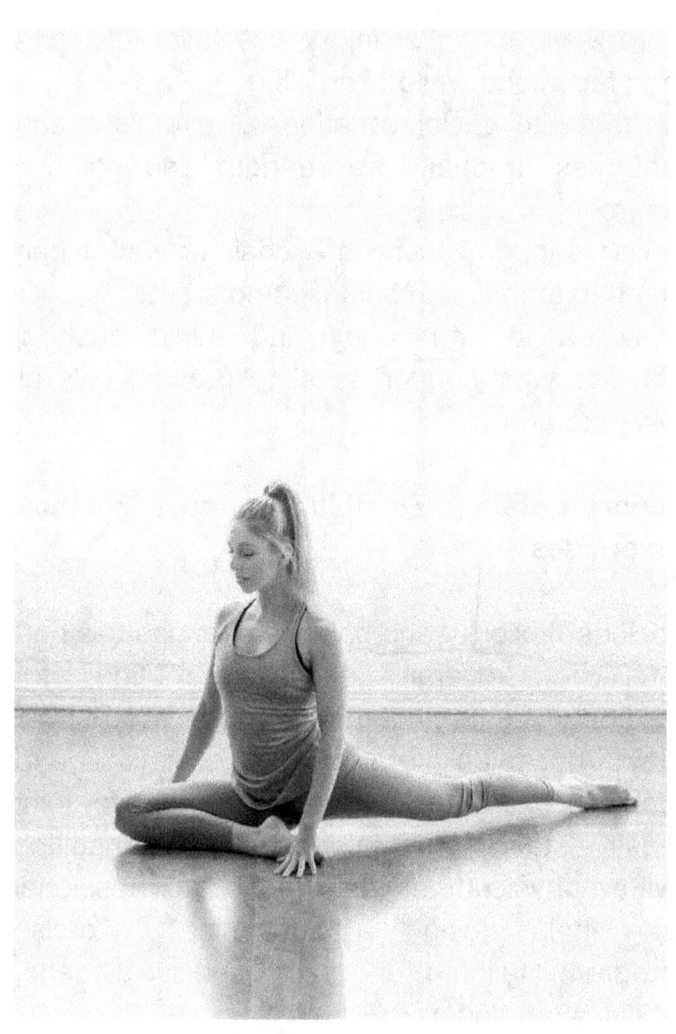

Chapter 6: Tailored Workout Plans

Tailoring a workout plan specifically for osteoporosis involves incorporating a combination of weight-bearing exercises, resistance training, flexibility exercises, and balance exercises to promote bone health, muscle strength, balance, and overall well-being. Here's how to create a tailored workout plan for osteoporosis management:

1.   **Consultation with Healthcare Professional**:

Before embarking on any exercise program, particularly for osteoporosis management, it is important to contact with a healthcare professional, such as a physical therapist or exercise physiologist.They can assess your bone health, physical capabilities, medical history, and any specific concerns to create a personalized workout plan that suits your needs.

2. **Key Components of a Personalized Workout Plan for Osteoporosis**:

-     Weight-Bearing Exercises: Include weight-bearing activities that involve impact or resistance on bones, such as walking, jogging, hiking, dancing, stair climbing, and aerobics. On most days of the week, aim for at least 30 minutes.

- Resistance Training: Incorporate resistance exercises using weights, resistance bands, or bodyweight exercises (like squats, lunges, push-ups) to build muscle strength and support bone health.
Perform resistance workouts 2-3 times each week.

- Flexibility Exercises: Include stretching routines for major muscle groups to improve joint mobility, reduce stiffness, and prevent injuries. Yoga, Pilates, and stretching exercises can enhance flexibility and relaxation.

- Balance and Stability Exercises: Incorporate balance exercises like single-leg stands, heel-to-toe walks, balance board exercises, and Tai Chi movements to improve balance, coordination, and reduce fall risk.

3. **Gradual Progression and Adaptation:**

- Start with low-impact exercises and gradually increase intensity, duration, and resistance as fitness improves.
- Monitor progress, listen to your body, and modify exercises as needed based on comfort, safety, and effectiveness.
- Add variation to your workout routine to target different muscle groups, avoid boredom, and improve overall fitness.

4. **Safety Tips and Precautions**:

- Practice proper form and technique during exercises to avoid strain or injury.
- Warm up before exercise and cool down afterward to prepare muscles and joints.
- Use appropriate footwear with good support and cushioning for weight-bearing activities.
- Stay hydrated, take breaks as needed, and listen to your body's signals during workouts.
- Avoid high-impact activities or movements that may increase fracture risk, especially if you have severe osteoporosis or other health concerns.

5. **Monitor and Adjust**:

- Regularly monitor your progress, symptoms, and any changes in bone health or fitness levels.
- Adjust your workout plan as needed based on feedback from healthcare professionals, personal goals, and individual capabilities.
- Be consistent with your exercise routine to maintain the benefits for bone health, muscle strength, balance, and overall well-being.

Sample Tailored Workout Plan for Osteoporosis:

1. Monday, Wednesday, Friday:
   - Warm-up (5-10 minutes of light cardio)
   - Resistance Training (2-3 sets of squats, lunges, chest presses, rows, and core exercises)
   - Flexibility Exercises (10-15 minutes of stretching focusing on major muscle groups)
   - Cool Down (5-10 minutes of gentle stretching)

2. Tuesday, Thursday, Saturday:
   - Warm-up (5-10 minutes of light cardio)
   - Weight-Bearing Exercises (30 minutes of brisk walking, dancing, or aerobics)

- Balance and Stability Exercises (10-15 minutes of single-leg stands, heel-to-toe walks, balance board exercises, or Tai Chi movements)
- Cool Down (5-10 minutes of gentle stretching)

3. Sunday:
- Rest day or light activity like gentle stretching, yoga, or leisurely walking.

This sample workout plan can be adjusted based on individual preferences, fitness level, and specific recommendations from healthcare providers. Consistency, progression, and proper technique are key to maximizing the benefits of exercise for osteoporosis management.

Beginner's Exercise Routine:

A beginner's exercise routine for osteoporosis should focus on gradual progression, safety, and effectiveness in improving bone health, muscle strength, balance, and overall fitness. It's important to start slowly, listen to your body, and consult with a healthcare professional before beginning any new exercise program. Here's a sample beginner's exercise routine for osteoporosis:

1. Warm-up (5-10 minutes):
   - Start with light cardio activities such as walking, marching in place, or cycling on a stationary bike.
   - Perform dynamic stretches to warm up major muscle groups, focusing on arms, legs, back, and core.

2. Weight-Bearing Exercises (15-20 minutes):
   - Begin with low-impact weight-bearing activities such as brisk walking, hiking on flat terrain, or using a treadmill with incline settings.
   - Aim for at least 10-15 minutes of continuous activity, gradually increasing duration as fitness improves.

3. Resistance Training (10-15 minutes):
   - Perform bodyweight exercises or use light resistance bands or dumbbells.
   - Examples include squats, lunges, wall push-ups, seated rows, and bicep curls.
   - Start with 1-2 sets of 8-12 repetitions for each exercise, focusing on proper form and controlled movements.

4. Flexibility and Stretching (10 minutes):
   - Incorporate static stretches for main muscle groups, holding each stretch for 15 to 30 seconds.
   - Include stretches for calves, quadriceps, hamstrings, hips, chest, shoulders, and back.
   - Use a yoga mat or comfortable surface for stretching exercises.

5. Balance and Stability Exercises (5-10 minutes):
   - Practice balance exercises to improve stability and reduce fall risk.
   - Examples include standing on one leg, heel-to-toe walking, and using a balance board or stability disc.
   - Use a sturdy chair or wall for support if needed, gradually increasing difficulty as balance improves.

6. Cool Down and Relaxation (5-10 minutes):
   - Conclude the workout with gentle cooling down activities such as walking at a slower pace or performing light stretching.
   - Incorporate deep breathing and relaxation techniques to promote stress reduction and recovery.

Important Tips for Beginners:
- Start with exercises that are comfortable and manageable, gradually increasing intensity, duration, and difficulty over time.
- Focus on proper form and technique during exercises to prevent injuries and maximize benefits.
- Listen to your body and maintain within what's comfortable for you.If you encounter pain or discomfort, stop exercising and seek medical attention.
- Stay hydrated and drink water before, during, and after exercise sessions.
- Incorporate variety into your routine to keep it interesting and enjoyable.
- Aim for consistency by planning regular workouts throughout the week.

Sample Beginner's Exercise Routine for Osteoporosis (30-40 minutes):

- Warm-up: 5 minutes of brisk walking or light cardio.
- Weight-Bearing Exercises: 15 minutes of walking or using a treadmill with incline settings.
- Resistance Training: 10 minutes of bodyweight exercises like squats, lunges, and wall push-ups.

- Flexibility and Stretching: 10 minutes of static stretching for major muscle groups.
- Balance and Stability Exercises: 5 minutes of balance exercises like standing on one leg and heel-to-toe walking.
- Cool Down and Relaxation: 5 minutes of gentle walking and deep breathing exercises.

Remember to improve gradually, remain consistent with your workouts, and adjust your schedule based on your specific needs and skills. If you have any health concerns or specific limitations, consult with a healthcare professional or physical therapist for personalized guidance.

Intermediate and Advanced Workouts:

For individuals with osteoporosis looking to progress beyond beginner-level workouts, intermediate and advanced exercise routines can provide additional challenges while still prioritizing bone health, muscle strength, balance, and overall fitness. Here are guidelines and examples for intermediate and advanced workouts tailored for osteoporosis management:

Intermediate Workout for Osteoporosis:

1. Warm-up (5-10 minutes):
   - Begin with light cardio activities such as brisk walking, cycling, or using an elliptical machine to increase heart rate and warm up muscles.
   - Include dynamic stretches for major muscle groups to improve flexibility and mobility.

2. Weight-Bearing Exercises (20-30 minutes):
   - Progress to moderate-intensity weight-bearing activities like jogging, hiking on varied terrain, or using a stair climber.
   - Aim for 15-20 minutes of continuous activity, gradually increasing intensity and duration as fitness improves.

3. Resistance Training (15-20 minutes):
   - Incorporate resistance exercises using moderate weights or resistance bands.
   - Include exercises like squats, lunges with weights, chest presses, rows, shoulder presses, and tricep dips.
   - Perform 2-3 sets of 10-12 repetitions for each exercise, focusing on proper form and controlled movements.

4. Flexibility and Stretching (10-15 minutes):

- Perform static stretches for major muscle groups, holding each stretch for 20-30 seconds to improve flexibility and reduce muscle tension.

- Include stretches for calves, quadriceps, hamstrings, hips, chest, shoulders, and back.

5. Balance and Stability Exercises (10-15 minutes):

- Integrate balance exercises such as single-leg stands, heel-to-toe walks, and using a balance board or stability disc to improve balance and coordination.

- Include exercises that challenge stability and proprioception without compromising safety.

6. Cool Down and Relaxation (5-10 minutes):

- Conclude the workout with gentle cool-down activities like walking at a slower pace and performing static stretches to promote relaxation and recovery.

Advanced Workout for Osteoporosis:

1. Warm-up (5-10 minutes):

- Begin with a dynamic warm-up including high knees, butt kicks, arm swings, and leg swings to prepare muscles and joints for intense activity.

- Incorporate mobility drills and foam rolling to improve range of motion and reduce muscle stiffness.

2. Weight-Bearing Exercises (30-45 minutes):

- Engage in high-intensity weight-bearing activities such as running, sprint intervals, plyometric exercises, or high-intensity interval training (HIIT) workouts.

- Alternate between periods of high intensity and recovery, challenging cardiovascular fitness and bone health.

3. Resistance Training (20-30 minutes):

- Use heavy weights or resistance bands with progressive overload to challenge muscle strength and bone density.

- Include compound exercises like deadlifts, squats with barbell, bench presses, pull-ups, and overhead presses.

- Perform 3-4 sets of 6-8 repetitions for each exercise, focusing on maximal effort and proper form.

4. Flexibility and Stretching (10-15 minutes):

- Incorporate dynamic stretching and mobility exercises as part of the warm-up and cool-down to improve flexibility and joint mobility.

- Include advanced yoga or Pilates poses for flexibility, strength, and balance.

5. Balance and Stability Exercises (15-20 minutes):

- Challenge balance and stability with advanced exercises such as single-leg squats with weights, bosu ball exercises, and agility drills.

- Incorporate multi-planar movements and functional exercises to simulate real-life activities and improve overall stability.

6. Cool Down and Recovery (10-15 minutes):

- Conclude the workout with a thorough cool-down including low-intensity activities like walking, gentle stretching, and foam rolling to aid in muscle recovery and relaxation.

- Practice deep breathing, meditation, or mindfulness techniques for stress reduction and mental recovery.

Important Considerations:

- Gradually progress from intermediate to advanced workouts based on individual fitness level, strength, and endurance.

- Focus on proper form, technique, and safety precautions to prevent injuries, especially for individuals with osteoporosis.
- Stay hydrated, fuel your body with nutritious foods, and prioritize adequate rest and recovery for optimal performance and recovery.
- Listen to your body's signals and adjust exercise intensity or volume as needed to avoid overtraining or fatigue.
- Consult with a healthcare professional or fitness expert for personalized guidance and recommendations, especially if you have osteoporosis or other health concerns.

By incorporating a balanced and progressive approach to exercise, individuals with osteoporosis can continue to improve bone health, muscle strength, balance, and overall fitness levels, leading to a healthier and more active lifestyle.

Incorporating Exercise into Daily Life:

Incorporating exercise into daily life for individuals with osteoporosis is crucial for improving bone health, muscle strength, balance, and overall well-being. By integrating physical activity into daily routines, it becomes easier to maintain consistency and achieve long-term health benefits. Here are practical tips for incorporating exercise into daily life for osteoporosis management:

1. Set Realistic Goals:
   - Start by setting realistic and achievable exercise goals based on your current fitness level, health status, and lifestyle.
   - Aim for at least 150 minutes of moderate-intensity aerobic activity or 75 minutes of vigorous-intensity aerobic activity every week, in accordance with health guidelines.

2.. Choose Activities You Enjoy:
   - Select physical activities that you enjoy and find enjoyable, whether it's walking, dancing, gardening, swimming, cycling, or group fitness classes.
   - Variety keeps exercise interesting and increases adherence to a regular routine.

3. Break Exercise into Short Sessions:
   - If time is limited, break exercise sessions into shorter bouts throughout the day. Aim for a minimum of 10 minutes of activity at a time.

- Incorporate activities like taking the stairs, walking during lunch breaks, or doing household chores that involve physical effort.

4. Make Exercise a Priority:
   - Schedule exercise sessions into your daily or weekly calendar, treating them as non-negotiable appointments.
   - Prioritize physical activity by finding ways to reduce sedentary time, such as standing breaks, stretching breaks, or active sitting options.

5. Integrate Exercise into Daily Tasks:
   - Walk or bike to nearby destinations instead of driving whenever possible.
   - Use a pedometer or fitness tracker to monitor daily steps and motivate movement.
   - Perform bodyweight exercises like squats, lunges, or wall push-ups during TV commercial breaks or while waiting for meals to cook.

6. Involve Family and Friends:
   - Encourage family members or friends to join you in physical activities, making exercise a social and enjoyable experience.
   - Plan active outings or recreational activities together, such as hiking, swimming, or playing sports.

7. Incorporate Strength Training:
- Include resistance exercises using bodyweight, resistance bands, or light weights into your routine to build muscle strength and support bone health.
- Perform strength training exercises 2-3 times a week, focusing on key muscle groups.

8. Prioritize Balance and Flexibility:
- Practice balance exercises like standing on one leg or heel-to-toe walking daily to improve stability and reduce fall risk.
- Incorporate flexibility exercises such as stretching or yoga to enhance joint mobility and reduce stiffness.

9. Monitor Progress and Adjust:
- Keep track of your exercise progress, noting improvements in strength, endurance, balance, and overall fitness.
- Adjust your exercise routine as needed based on feedback from your body, health professionals, or changes in health status.

10. Stay Consistent and Be Patient:
- Consistency is key to reaping the benefits of exercise for osteoporosis management.

Stick to your exercise routine even on days when motivation is low.

- Be patient with your progress, as improvements in bone health and fitness take time and dedication.

11. Listen to Your Body:

- Pay attention to how your body reacts to exercise. If you experience pain or discomfort, modify activities or seek guidance from a healthcare professional.

- Stay hydrated, practice good nutrition, and get adequate rest for optimal recovery and overall health.

By incorporating exercise into daily life and making it a regular habit, individuals with osteoporosis can improve bone health, muscle strength, balance, and overall quality of life. Consistency, variety, and enjoyment are key factors in maintaining an active and healthy lifestyle.

Part III: Natural Remedies:

Natural remedies can complement medical treatments and lifestyle changes for managing osteoporosis. While they may not replace conventional therapies, they can contribute to overall bone health and well-being. Here are some natural remedies and lifestyle interventions that may benefit individuals with osteoporosis:

1. **Dietary Changes**:
   - Calcium-Rich Foods: Include dairy products (low-fat milk, yogurt, cheese), leafy green vegetables (kale, spinach, broccoli), almonds, and fortified foods in your diet to support bone strength.
   - Vitamin D Sources: Get adequate sunlight exposure and consume foods rich in vitamin D such as fatty fish (salmon, mackerel), egg yolks, fortified cereals, and supplements if needed for optimal bone health.
   - Magnesium and Vitamin K: Incorporate magnesium-rich foods (nuts, seeds, whole grains) and vitamin K-rich foods (leafy

greens, broccoli, Brussels sprouts) to support bone mineralization and density.

- Omega-3 Fatty Acids: Include sources of omega-3 fatty acids such as fish oil, flaxseeds, chia seeds, and walnuts to reduce inflammation and support bone health.

2. **Herbal Remedies**:

- Horsetail Herb: Contains silica, which is important for bone health and collagen formation. It is available in tea or supplement form but should be used cautiously and under supervision due to potential side effects.

- Red Clover: Contains isoflavones that may help maintain bone density. It can be consumed as tea or in supplement form but consult with a healthcare provider before use, especially for individuals with hormone-related conditions.

- Black Cohosh: Some studies suggest that black cohosh may have bone-protective effects, particularly in postmenopausal women. It is available as a supplement but should be used with caution and under supervision.

3. **Regular Physical Activity**:
    - Engage in weight-bearing exercises such as walking, jogging, dancing, stair climbing, and resistance training to promote bone strength and density.
    - Include balance exercises and activities that improve posture and coordination to reduce the risk of falls and fractures.
    - Indulge in flexibility exercises like yoga or Pilates to maintain joint mobility and reduce stiffness.

4. **Maintain a Healthy Weight**:
    - Aim for a healthy weight to reduce strain on bones and joints. Avoid extreme dieting or rapid weight loss, as it can lead to bone loss.
    - Incorporate a balanced diet rich in nutrients essential for bone health, and avoid excessive alcohol consumption and smoking, which can negatively impact bone density.

5. **Limit Caffeine and Sodium Intake**:
    - Excessive caffeine and sodium intake can contribute to calcium loss from bones.

Limit consumption of coffee, tea, soda, and processed foods high in sodium.

6. **Mind-Body Practices**:
   - Manage stress through relaxation techniques such as deep breathing, meditation, tai chi, or yoga, as chronic stress can affect bone health and overall well-being.

7. **Supplements (Under Supervision):**
   - Consider supplements such as calcium, vitamin D, magnesium, and vitamin K under the guidance of a healthcare professional, especially if dietary intake is insufficient.
   - Avoid excessive supplementation and be cautious with herbal remedies, as they may interact with medications or have side effects.

8. **Regular Bone Density Monitoring**:
   - Follow up with healthcare providers for regular bone density tests (DEXA scans) to monitor bone health and assess the effectiveness of interventions.

It's essential to consult with a healthcare provider or a registered dietitian before starting any new supplements or herbal remedies, especially if you have underlying health conditions or are taking medications. Integrating these natural remedies with a comprehensive treatment plan, including medication, exercise, and dietary changes, can support optimal bone health and management of osteoporosis.

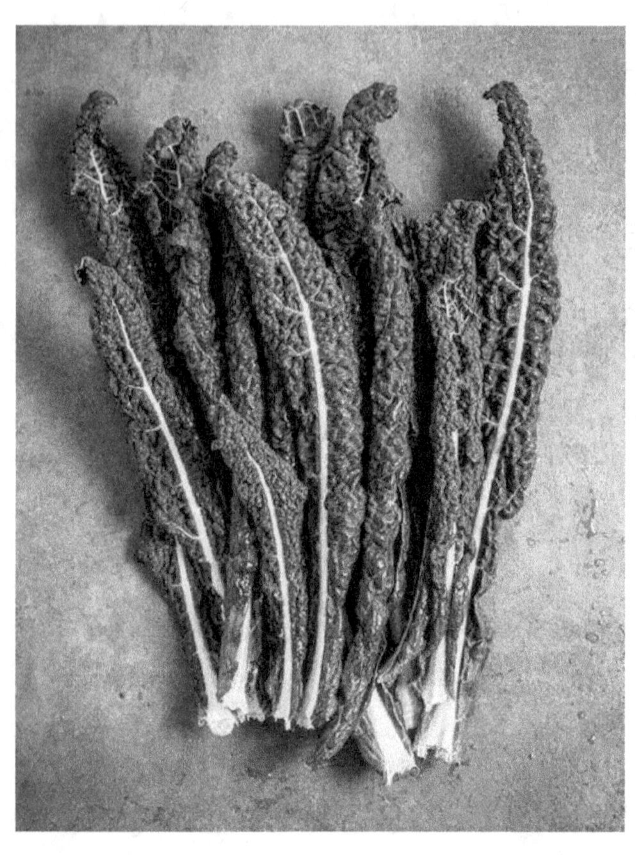

Chapter 7: Herbal and Nutritional Supplements

Herbal and nutritional supplements can be valuable additions to a comprehensive osteoporosis management plan. However, it's crucial to use them cautiously and under the guidance of a healthcare professional, as they may interact with medications or have side effects. Here are some herbal and nutritional supplements commonly used for osteoporosis:

1. **Calcium Supplements**:
   - Calcium is essential for bone health, and many individuals with osteoporosis may require supplements to meet their daily calcium needs.
   - Calcium supplements are available in various forms, such as calcium carbonate and calcium citrate. For optimal absorption, take with a meal. Excessive calcium intake is not recommended, as it might cause constipation or kidney stones.

2. **Vitamin D Supplements**:
   - Vitamin D is essential for calcium absorption and bone health. Many people,

especially those with limited sun exposure, may require vitamin D supplementation.

- Vitamin D supplements are available in different strengths (e.g., vitamin D2 and vitamin D3). The preferred form for supplementation is usually vitamin D3 (cholecalciferol).

- Healthcare providers may recommend specific dosages based on individual needs and blood test results.

3. **Magnesium Supplements**:

- Magnesium plays a role in bone mineralization and is important for overall bone health.

- Magnesium supplements can be beneficial for individuals with low magnesium levels or those who have difficulty obtaining enough magnesium from their diet.

- Dosage recommendations vary depending on age, gender, and health status. Excessive magnesium intake can cause gastrointestinal symptoms.

4. **Vitamin K Supplements**:

- Vitamin K is involved in bone metabolism and helps activate proteins that regulate calcium in bones.

- Vitamin K supplements, particularly vitamin K2 (menaquinone), may support bone density and reduce fracture risk.

- Individuals taking blood-thinning medications (anticoagulants) should consult their healthcare provider before taking vitamin K supplements.

5. **Herbal Supplements**:

- Horsetail (Equisetum arvense): Horsetail contains silica, which is important for collagen formation and bone health. It may be available in supplement form or used as a tea.

- Red Clover (Trifolium pratense): Red clover contains isoflavones that may have bone-protective effects. It can be taken as a supplement or in the form of herbal tea.

- Black Cohosh (Actaea racemosa): Some studies suggest that black cohosh may support bone density, especially in postmenopausal women. It is available as a supplement.

6. **Omega-3 Fatty Acids**:

- Omega-3 fatty acids, found in fish oil supplements, flaxseeds, and walnuts, have anti-inflammatory properties and may support bone health indirectly by reducing inflammation.

- Fish oil supplements are a common source of omega-3s, but they should be used cautiously, especially in individuals taking blood-thinning medications.

7. **Collagen Supplements**:
   - Collagen is a protein found in bones, skin, and connective tissues. Collagen supplements may promote bone health and joint function.
   - Collagen supplements are available in various forms, including collagen peptides and hydrolyzed collagen. They are often marketed for joint and bone support.

8. **Probiotics**:
   - Probiotics are beneficial bacteria that support gut health and may indirectly impact bone health by enhancing nutrient absorption and immune function.
   - Certain strains of probiotics, such as Lactobacillus and Bifidobacterium species, have been studied for their potential role in bone metabolism.

It's important to note that while these supplements may offer potential benefits for osteoporosis, they should not replace a balanced diet, regular exercise, and medical treatments prescribed by healthcare providers.

Before starting any supplements, discuss your individual needs, medical history, and potential interactions with medications with a healthcare professional or registered dietitian. They can help determine the appropriate dosage, form, and duration of supplementation based on your specific health goals and concerns. Regular monitoring and follow-up are essential to assess the effectiveness and safety of herbal and nutritional supplements for osteoporosis management.

Benefits of Herbal Remedies:

Herbal remedies are often sought as complementary or alternative approaches to managing osteoporosis. While research on their efficacy is ongoing, several herbal remedies have shown potential benefits for bone health and osteoporosis management. Here are some of the potential benefits of herbal remedies for osteoporosis:

1. **Support Bone Density**:
   - Certain herbs contain compounds that may support bone density and strength. For

example, herbs like horsetail (Equisetum arvense) and red clover (Trifolium pratense) are rich in minerals like silica and isoflavones, respectively, which are believed to contribute to bone health.

2. **Anti-Inflammatory Properties**:

- Many herbal remedies possess anti-inflammatory properties, which can be beneficial for individuals with osteoporosis. Chronic inflammation is linked to bone loss, and herbs like turmeric (Curcuma longa) and ginger (Zingiber officinale) have been studied for their anti-inflammatory effects.

3. **Hormonal Balance**:

- Some herbs, such as black cohosh (Actaea racemosa), may help balance hormones, particularly in postmenopausal women. Hormonal changes can affect bone density, and herbs that support hormonal balance may indirectly benefit bone health.

4. **Antioxidant Activity**:

- Several herbs are rich in antioxidants, which can protect cells from damage and promote overall health. Antioxidants may play a role in reducing oxidative stress and supporting bone health.

5. **Collagen Production**:
   - Collagen is a protein essential for bone structure and strength. Some herbs, such as gotu kola (Centella asiatica) and horsetail, are believed to support collagen production, which may benefit bone health.

6. **Calcium Absorption**:
   - Certain herbs, when consumed as part of a balanced diet, may enhance calcium absorption. For example, nettle leaf (Urtica dioica) is a nutrient-rich herb that contains minerals like calcium and magnesium, which are important for bone health.

7. **Improved Digestion and Nutrient Absorption**:
   - Herbal remedies that support digestive health, such as ginger, peppermint (Mentha piperita), and fennel (Foeniculum vulgare), can improve nutrient absorption, including minerals essential for bone health.

8. **Stress Reduction**:
   - Chronic stress can reduce bone density. Adaptogenic herbs like ashwagandha (Withania somnifera) and holy basil (Ocimum

sanctum) may help reduce stress levels, potentially benefiting bone health indirectly.

9. **Safe and Natural Approach**:
   - Herbal remedies are often perceived as safer and more natural alternatives to pharmaceutical medications. When used appropriately and under professional guidance, herbal remedies can be integrated into a holistic approach to osteoporosis management.

10. **Complementary to Conventional Treatments:**
   - Herbal remedies can complement conventional treatments for osteoporosis, such as medication, exercise, and dietary changes. They may provide additional support for bone health and overall well-being.

It's important to note that while herbal remedies offer potential benefits, they should not replace evidence-based medical treatments or lifestyle modifications recommended by healthcare providers. Before using herbal remedies for osteoporosis, consult with a qualified healthcare professional or herbalist to determine the most appropriate herbs, dosages, and potential interactions with medications. Individual responses to herbal remedies may vary, and regular monitoring is essential to assess their effectiveness and safety.

Supplementing Calcium and Vitamin D:

Supplementing with calcium and vitamin D is a common and essential part of managing osteoporosis. Both nutrients play crucial roles in bone health, and their supplementation can help support bone density, strength, and overall skeletal integrity. Here's a detailed look at supplementing calcium and vitamin D for osteoporosis:

1. **Calcium Supplementation**:

- Role in Bone Health: Calcium is a vital mineral that makes up a significant portion of bone tissue. Adequate calcium consumption are crucial for keeping strong and healthy bones.

- Daily Requirements: The recommended daily intake of calcium varies based on age, sex, and other factors. For adults, the general guideline is around 1000-1200 milligrams per day.

- Calcium Sources: Dietary sources of calcium include dairy products (milk, yogurt, cheese), fortified plant-based milk alternatives, green leafy vegetables (kale, spinach), tofu, almonds, and sardines with bones.

- Supplementation Considerations: Calcium supplements are available in various forms, such as calcium carbonate and calcium citrate. Calcium carbonate should be taken with meals for optimal absorption, while calcium citrate can be taken with or without food.

- Combination Supplements: Some calcium supplements also contain vitamin D, magnesium, or other minerals that support bone health. Combination supplements can be convenient for individuals who need multiple nutrients for bone support.

- Potential Side Effects: Excessive calcium intake from supplements may lead to side effects such as constipation, bloating, and kidney stones. It's important to follow recommended dosages and consult with a healthcare professional before starting calcium supplementation.

2. Vitamin D Supplementation:

- Role in Bone Health: Vitamin D is crucial for calcium absorption and utilization in the body. It helps maintain proper calcium levels in the blood and supports bone mineralization.

- Sources of Vitamin D: The primary source of vitamin D is sunlight exposure, which triggers vitamin D synthesis in the skin. Dietary sources include fatty fish (salmon, mackerel), egg yolks, fortified foods (milk, cereals, orange juice), and vitamin D supplements.

- Daily Requirements: The recommended daily intake of vitamin D varies by age, with adults typically needing around 600-800 international units (IU) per day. However, individual needs may vary based on factors like sun exposure and health status.

- Supplementation Benefits: Many people, especially those with limited sun exposure or certain medical conditions, may benefit from vitamin D supplementation. It can help maintain adequate vitamin D levels in the body, which is important for bone health.

- Types of Vitamin D Supplements: Vitamin D supplements are available in two main forms: vitamin D2 (ergocalciferol) and vitamin D3 (cholecalciferol). Vitamin D3 is considered more effective at raising blood levels of vitamin D and is the preferred form for supplementation.

- Optimal Blood Levels: Healthcare providers may assess vitamin D levels through blood tests (25-hydroxyvitamin D). Optimal blood levels of vitamin D for bone health are generally considered to be between 30-50 nanograms per milliliter (ng/mL).

- Combination Supplements: Some calcium supplements come in combination with vitamin D, which can be beneficial for individuals who need both nutrients for bone support.

Important Considerations:
1. Consultation with Healthcare Provider: Before starting calcium or vitamin D supplementation, it's crucial to consult with a healthcare provider. They can assess your individual needs, recommend appropriate

dosages, and monitor your response to supplementation.

2. Monitoring Calcium Intake: Be mindful of your total calcium intake from both dietary sources and supplements. Excessive calcium intake can lead to health issues, so it's important to stay within recommended limits.

3. Sun Exposure: While sunlight is a natural source of vitamin D, factors like geographic location, season, skin pigmentation, and sunscreen use can affect vitamin D synthesis. Individuals with limited sun exposure may require supplementation.

4. Adherence to Guidelines: Follow recommended guidelines for calcium and vitamin D supplementation, and avoid self-prescribing high doses without professional guidance.

5. Potential Interactions: Some medications and health conditions may interact with calcium or vitamin D supplements. Inform your healthcare provider about all medications, supplements, and health concerns before starting supplementation.

Supplementing with calcium and vitamin D, along with a balanced diet, regular exercise, and other lifestyle modifications, can significantly contribute to the management of osteoporosis and support overall bone health. However, individual needs may vary, so personalized guidance from a healthcare provider is essential for safe and effective supplementation.

Safety and Precautions:

Safety and precautions are essential considerations for individuals with osteoporosis to prevent fractures, minimize risks, and maintain overall well-being. Here are important safety measures and precautions to follow when managing osteoporosis:

1. **Regular Medical Check-ups:**
   - Schedule regular check-ups with your healthcare provider to monitor bone density, assess fracture risk, and review treatment effectiveness.
   - Follow recommended guidelines for bone density testing (DEXA scans) based on age, risk factors, and medical history.

2. **Medication Adherence:**

- Take the recommended medications as directed by your healthcare provider. Follow dosage instructions, and inform your doctor about any side effects or concerns.

- Do not stop using or change drugs without consulting your doctor.

3. **Fall Prevention:**

- Create a safe environment at home by removing tripping hazards, securing rugs, and installing handrails and grab bars in bathrooms and stairways.

- Use non-slip mats in the bathroom, and ensure adequate lighting in all areas of the house, especially at night.

- Wear appropriate footwear with good traction to prevent slips and falls.

4. **Balance and Strength Training:**

- Engage in regular physical activity, including exercises that improve balance, strength, and flexibility.

- Consider working with a physical therapist to develop a personalized exercise plan tailored to your needs and abilities.

- Use caution when performing activities that may increase fall risk, such as climbing ladders or walking on icy surfaces.

5. **Proper Body Mechanics**:

- Practice proper body mechanics to avoid strain on your spine and joints. Use correct lifting techniques, bend at the knees when lifting objects, and avoid twisting motions.

- Use assistive devices like a walker or cane if needed for stability and support.

6. **Nutrition and Hydration**:

- Follow a balanced diet rich in calcium, vitamin D, magnesium, and other essential nutrients for bone health.

- Stay hydrated by drinking an adequate amount of water daily, as dehydration can affect muscle function and balance.

7. **Avoid Smoking and Limit Alcohol**:

- Smoking and excessive alcohol consumption can weaken bones and increase fracture risk. Quit smoking, and limit alcohol intake to promote bone health.

8. **Bone Health Supplements**:

- If recommended by your healthcare provider, take calcium, vitamin D, and other bone-supporting supplements as prescribed. Avoid excessive supplementation without professional guidance.

9. **Regular Vision and Hearing Checks**:

- Maintain regular vision and hearing checks, as impaired vision or hearing can contribute to falls and accidents.

10. **Medication Review**:

- Review all medications with your healthcare provider, including over-the-counter drugs and supplements, to identify any potential interactions or side effects that may impact bone health or fall risk.

11. **Bone Density Monitoring**:

- Follow up with bone density testing as recommended by your healthcare provider to track changes in bone health and assess fracture risk.

12. **Educate Yourself:**

- Stay informed about osteoporosis, its management, and preventive measures. Attend educational workshops, read reputable sources, and ask questions during medical appointments.

13. **Emergency Preparedness**:

- Have a plan in place for emergencies, including knowing how to contact emergency services, keeping a list of medications and medical conditions handy, and having emergency contact information readily available.

By following these safety precautions and guidelines, individuals with osteoporosis can reduce the risk of fractures, improve overall bone health, and enhance quality of life. It's important to work closely with healthcare providers, adhere to treatment plans, and make lifestyle adjustments to manage osteoporosis effectively.

Chapter 8: Lifestyle Modifications

Lifestyle modifications play a crucial role in managing osteoporosis and reducing the risk of fractures. By adopting healthy habits and making targeted lifestyle changes, individuals with osteoporosis can support bone health, improve overall well-being, and minimize complications. Here are key lifestyle modifications for osteoporosis management:

1. **Nutritious Diet**:
   - Calcium-Rich Foods: Include dairy products (low-fat milk, yogurt, cheese), leafy green vegetables (kale, spinach, broccoli), almonds, and fortified foods in your diet to meet calcium needs for bone health.
   - Vitamin D Sources: Get adequate sunlight exposure and consume foods rich in vitamin D such as fatty fish (salmon, mackerel), egg yolks, fortified cereals, and supplements if needed for optimal bone health.
   - Magnesium and Vitamin K: Incorporate magnesium-rich foods (nuts, seeds, whole grains) and vitamin K-rich foods (leafy greens,

broccoli, Brussels sprouts) to support bone mineralization and density.

- Protein: Consume adequate protein from lean meats, poultry, fish, legumes, and plant-based sources to support muscle strength and overall health.

- Limit Sodium and Caffeine: Reduce consumption of salty foods and beverages high in caffeine, as excessive intake can contribute to calcium loss from bones.

2. **Regular Exercise**:

- Weight-Bearing Exercises: Engage in weight-bearing activities such as walking, jogging, hiking, dancing, stair climbing, and resistance training to strengthen bones and improve balance.

- Strength Training: Include resistance exercises using bodyweight, free weights, or resistance bands to build muscle strength and support bone density.

- Balance and Flexibility Exercises: Practice balance exercises such as standing on one leg, heel-to-toe walking, and yoga or tai chi to improve balance, stability, and coordination.

- Posture Improvement: Maintain good posture during daily activities and use proper body mechanics to reduce strain on the spine and joints.

3. **Fall Prevention**:
   - Create a safe home environment by removing tripping hazards, securing rugs, installing handrails and grab bars, and ensuring adequate lighting.
   - Use assistive devices like a cane or walker if needed for stability and support.
   - Wear supportive footwear with good traction to prevent slips and falls.

4. **Healthy Lifestyle Choices**:
   - Quit Smoking: Smoking can weaken bones and increase fracture risk. Quit smoking to improve bone health and overall well-being.
   - Limit Alcohol: Excessive alcohol consumption can negatively impact bone density. Limit alcohol intake to promote bone health.
   - Maintain a Healthy Weight: Aim for a healthy weight to reduce strain on bones and joints. Avoid extreme dieting or rapid weight loss, as it can lead to bone loss.

5. **Bone Health Monitoring**:
   - Follow up with healthcare providers for regular bone density testing (DEXA scans) to monitor bone health, assess fracture risk, and evaluate the effectiveness of treatments.

- Discuss medication adherence, potential side effects, and any concerns with your healthcare team.

6. **Stress Management**:
   - Practice stress-reducing techniques such as deep breathing, meditation, yoga, or mindfulness to reduce stress levels, which can impact bone health.
   - Get adequate sleep and prioritize relaxation to support overall well-being.

7. **Education and Support**:
   - Stay informed about osteoporosis, its management, and preventive measures. Attend educational workshops, seek guidance from healthcare providers, and connect with support groups or resources for additional information and support.

By incorporating these lifestyle modifications into daily routines, individuals with osteoporosis can take proactive steps to support bone health, reduce fracture risk, and enhance overall quality of life. It's important to work closely with healthcare providers to develop a personalized plan that addresses individual needs and goals for osteoporosis management.

Stress Reduction Techniques:

Stress reduction techniques are valuable for individuals with osteoporosis as chronic stress can negatively impact bone health and overall well-being. By incorporating stress-reducing practices into daily life, individuals can promote relaxation, reduce tension, and support bone health. Here are effective stress reduction techniques for osteoporosis:

1. **Deep Breathing Exercises**:
   - To help you relax and cope with stress, try deep breathing techniques. Take a comfortable seat or lie down, close your eyes, and inhale deeply through your nose and exhale slowly through your mouth. Focus on expanding your abdomen with each inhale and releasing tension with each exhale.

2. **Mindfulness Meditation**:
   - Practice mindfulness meditation to develop present-moment awareness and lessen anxiety.
Find a quiet space, sit comfortably, and focus your attention on your breath, sensations in your body, or a calming mantra. Accept and

acknowledge your thoughts as they present themselves.

3. **Progressive Muscle Relaxation (PMR):**

- Practice progressive muscle relaxation by systematically tensing and releasing different muscle groups in your body. Start with your toes and work your way up to your head, focusing on each muscle group for a few seconds before relaxing completely.

4. **Yoga and Tai Chi:**

- Participate in yoga or tai chi classes, which combine gentle movements, deep breathing, and mindfulness to reduce stress, improve flexibility, and enhance overall well-being. Choose classes specifically designed for bone health if available.

5. **Guided Imagery and Visualization:**

- Use guided imagery or visualization techniques to create a mental image of a peaceful, calming place. Close your eyes, imagine yourself in this serene environment, and focus on the sensory details to evoke relaxation and reduce stress.

6. **Journaling and Expressive Writing**:
   - Keep a journal to express your thoughts, emotions, and experiences. Writing can be a therapeutic outlet for processing stress, identifying triggers, and gaining insights into your feelings.

7. **Physical Activity and Exercise**:
   - Engage in regular physical activity and exercise, such as walking, swimming, dancing, or cycling, to release endorphins (feel-good hormones) and reduce stress levels. Choose activities that you enjoy and can incorporate into your routine.

8. **Social Support and Connection**:
   - Stay connected with supportive friends, family members, or support groups. Share your feelings, seek advice, and engage in meaningful conversations to alleviate stress and build a sense of belonging.

9. **Healthy Lifestyle Habits**:
   - Maintain a balanced diet, get adequate sleep, and prioritize self-care practices like massage, aromatherapy, or relaxation baths with Epsom salts to promote relaxation and reduce stress.

10. **Professional Support**:

- Consider seeking support from mental health professionals, such as therapists or counselors, who can provide guidance, coping strategies, and tools for managing stress effectively.

It's important to integrate stress reduction techniques into your daily routine and practice consistency to experience long-term benefits. Experiment with different techniques to find what works best for you, and prioritize self-care to support overall well-being and bone health. Remember that reducing stress is a proactive step toward managing osteoporosis and improving quality of life.

Smoking and Alcohol Cessation:

Smoking and excessive alcohol consumption can have significant negative effects on bone health, exacerbating the risk of osteoporosis and fractures. Here's an overview of how smoking and alcohol cessation can impact osteoporosis:

1. **Smoking Cessation**:

- Bone Density Loss: Smoking is associated with reduced bone density and increased risk of fractures, particularly in the hip and spine. The harmful chemicals in tobacco smoke interfere with bone remodeling, leading to accelerated bone loss.

- Hormonal Disruption: Smoking can disrupt hormone levels, including estrogen in women and testosterone in men, which are essential for maintaining bone density. This hormonal imbalance contributes to bone weakening and osteoporosis.

- Inflammatory Response: Smoking triggers inflammation throughout the body, including in bone tissues. Chronic inflammation interferes with bone formation and repair processes, further compromising bone health.

- Impaired Calcium Absorption: Smoking interferes with the body's ability to absorb calcium, a crucial mineral for bone strength. This calcium imbalance contributes to weakened bones and increased fracture risk.

- Delayed Healing: Smokers may experience delayed bone healing and poorer outcomes after fractures or orthopedic surgeries due to impaired blood flow, reduced oxygen delivery, and compromised immune function.

- Benefits of Smoking Cessation: Quitting smoking can lead to significant improvements in bone health over time. Studies have shown that individuals who quit smoking experience slower rates of bone loss and reduced fracture risk compared to smokers.

2. **Alcohol Cessation**:

- Bone Density Reduction: Excessive alcohol consumption is linked to decreased bone density and increased risk of fractures. Alcohol disrupts bone formation and remodeling processes, leading to weaker bones.

- Nutrient Absorption Interference: Alcohol interferes with the absorption and utilization of essential nutrients for bone health, including calcium, vitamin D, magnesium, and vitamin K. This nutrient imbalance contributes to bone weakening.

- Hormonal Imbalance: Chronic alcohol abuse can disrupt hormone levels, such as reducing testosterone and estrogen production, which are important for maintaining bone density and strength.

- Liver Function: Prolonged alcohol consumption can impair liver function, leading to reduced vitamin D activation and metabolism. For the body to absorb calcium and for bones to mineralize, vitamin D is crucial.

- Increased Fall Risk: Alcohol consumption can impair coordination, balance, and judgment, increasing the risk of falls and fractures, especially in older adults.

- Benefits of Alcohol Cessation: Cutting back on alcohol or quitting altogether can help preserve bone density, reduce fracture risk, improve nutrient absorption, and support overall bone health.

By quitting smoking and moderating alcohol consumption, individuals can take proactive steps to protect their bones, reduce the risk of osteoporosis and fractures, and support overall health and well-being. It's important to seek support from healthcare professionals, counselors, or support groups if needed to successfully quit smoking or reduce alcohol intake.

Sleep and Bone Health:

Sleep plays a vital role in maintaining optimal bone health and preventing osteoporosis. The relationship between sleep and bone health is multifaceted, with various physiological processes influenced by sleep duration, quality, and patterns. Here's how sleep impacts bone health and its relation to osteoporosis:

1. **Bone Formation and Repair**:
   - During sleep, especially during deep sleep stages, the body undergoes crucial processes for bone formation and repair. Growth hormone (GH) and insulin-like growth factor 1 (IGF-1) are released during these stages, stimulating bone growth, development, and repair.
   - Adequate sleep duration and quality are essential for optimal production and activity of osteoblasts, the cells responsible for building new bone tissue. These cells synthesize collagen and other components necessary for bone strength and density.

2. **Hormonal Regulation:**

- Sleep influences the regulation of several hormones that play key roles in bone health. Growth hormone, as mentioned earlier, promotes bone growth and regeneration.

- Melatonin, a hormone primarily associated with sleep regulation, also contributes to bone health. It has antioxidant properties that protect bone cells from oxidative damage and supports bone mineral density.

3. **Calcium Metabolism:**

- Sleep affects calcium metabolism, a critical process for maintaining bone strength. Adequate sleep helps regulate parathyroid hormone (PTH) levels, which play a role in calcium absorption and utilization.

- Disrupted sleep patterns or sleep deprivation can lead to imbalances in calcium metabolism, potentially contributing to reduced bone density and increased bone resorption.

4. **Inflammatory Response:**

- Chronic sleep disturbances or insufficient sleep can trigger systemic inflammation, which negatively impacts bone health. Inflammation disrupts the balance between bone formation by osteoblasts and bone resorption by osteoclasts, leading to bone loss over time.

5. **Muscle Function and Balance:**

- Quality sleep supports muscle recovery, strength, and coordination, which are essential for maintaining balance and reducing the risk of falls and fractures.

- Strong muscles provide support to bones and help protect against fractures, especially in weight-bearing bones like the hips and spine.

6. **Sleep Disorders and Osteoporosis Risk:**

- Certain sleep disorders, such as sleep apnea, insomnia, and restless leg syndrome, have been linked to an increased risk of osteoporosis and fractures.

- Sleep apnea, characterized by interrupted breathing during sleep, may contribute to systemic inflammation and hormonal imbalances that affect bone health.

- Chronic insomnia or poor sleep quality can lead to elevated stress hormone levels (cortisol), which can promote bone breakdown and weaken bone structure over time.

7. **Lifestyle Factors:**

- Healthy sleep habits are often part of a broader lifestyle approach to bone health. Maintaining a regular sleep schedule, creating a sleep-conducive environment, and practicing relaxation techniques can positively impact both sleep quality and bone health.

- Combining good sleep hygiene with a balanced diet, regular exercise, and avoiding harmful habits like smoking and excessive alcohol consumption can further support overall bone health and reduce the risk of osteoporosis.

In conclusion, prioritizing healthy sleep habits is crucial for maintaining optimal bone health and reducing the risk of osteoporosis and fractures. Adequate sleep duration, quality, and patterns support bone formation, hormonal balance, calcium metabolism, and muscle function, all of which contribute to skeletal strength and resilience. Incorporating strategies for improving sleep hygiene into daily routines can have significant benefits for bone health and overall well-being.

Part IV: Bonus – Healthy Bone Recipes

Eating a balanced diet rich in nutrients essential for bone health is crucial for preventing osteoporosis and maintaining strong bones. Healthy bone recipes can incorporate ingredients high in calcium, vitamin D, magnesium, vitamin K, and other nutrients vital for bone strength and density. Here are some examples of healthy bone recipes along with their benefits for osteoporosis:

1. **Salmon and Spinach Salad:**

   - Ingredients: Grilled salmon fillet, fresh spinach leaves, cherry tomatoes, cucumber slices, avocado slices, walnuts, olive oil, lemon juice, salt, and pepper.
   - Benefits: Salmon is rich in omega-3 fatty acids, vitamin D, and protein, which support bone health and reduce inflammation. Spinach provides calcium, magnesium, and vitamin K necessary for bone strength. Walnuts offer additional omega-3s and antioxidants.

2. **Greek Yogurt Parfait:**

- Ingredients: Greek yogurt (plain or flavored), mixed berries (strawberries, blueberries, raspberries), granola, chia seeds, honey or maple syrup.

- Benefits: Greek yogurt is a good source of calcium, protein, and probiotics that aid in calcium absorption. Berries provide antioxidants, vitamins, and minerals that support overall health. Chia seeds add omega-3s and fiber.

3. **Quinoa and Vegetable Stir-Fry**:

- Ingredients: Cooked quinoa, mixed vegetables (bell peppers, broccoli, carrots, snap peas), tofu or chicken breast strips, garlic, ginger, soy sauce or tamari, sesame oil, sesame seeds.

- Benefits: Quinoa is a plant-based source of protein, calcium, magnesium, and fiber. Tofu (or chicken) adds protein and minerals. Vegetables offer vitamins, antioxidants, and phytonutrients that promote bone health.

4. **Kale and Chickpea Salad**:

- Ingredients: Chopped kale, cooked chickpeas, diced bell peppers, red onion, feta cheese (optional), olives, olive oil, lemon juice, Dijon mustard, salt, and pepper.

   - Benefits: Kale is a powerhouse of calcium, vitamin K, and antioxidants that support bone density. Chickpeas provide protein, fiber, and minerals like magnesium and phosphorus. Olive oil adds healthy fats, and lemon juice enhances vitamin C absorption.

5. Mushroom and Spinach Omelet:

   - Ingredients: Eggs, sliced mushrooms, fresh spinach leaves, onion, garlic, grated cheese (optional), olive oil, salt, and pepper.

   - **Benefits:** Eggs are a good source of vitamin D, protein, and minerals like phosphorus. Spinach contributes calcium, vitamin K, and magnesium. Mushrooms provide vitamin D when exposed to sunlight or UV light.

6. Baked Sweet Potato with Broccoli and Cottage Cheese:

   - Ingredients: Baked sweet potato, steamed broccoli florets, cottage cheese, chopped fresh herbs (parsley, chives), olive oil, salt, and pepper.

- Benefits: Sweet potatoes are rich in vitamin A, potassium, and fiber. Broccoli offers calcium, vitamin K, and antioxidants. Cottage cheese provides protein, calcium, and phosphorus for bone strength.

These healthy bone recipes are nutrient-dense, flavorful, and easy to prepare, making them excellent choices for supporting bone health and overall well-being, especially for individuals at risk of osteoporosis or seeking to maintain strong bones.

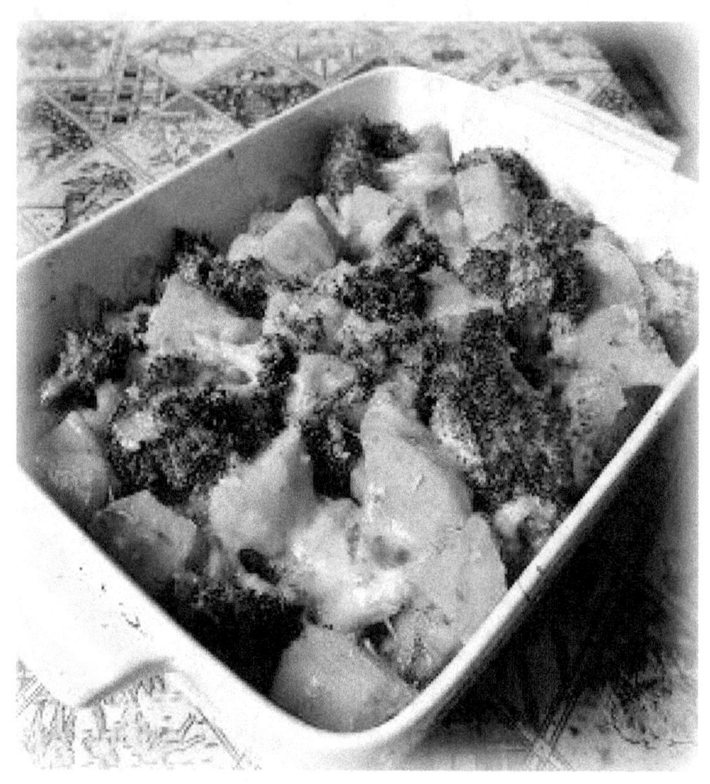

Chapter 9: Nutritious Recipes for Stronger Bones

Nutritious recipes tailored for stronger bones are essential for individuals managing osteoporosis or aiming to support bone health. These recipes focus on ingredients rich in calcium, vitamin D, magnesium, vitamin K, protein, and other nutrients crucial for maintaining bone density and strength. Here are some nutritious recipes designed specifically for stronger bones:

1. Creamy Spinach and Mushroom Pasta:

- **Ingredients**:
    - Whole wheat pasta
    - Fresh spinach leaves
    - Sliced mushrooms
    - Garlic cloves, minced
    - Olive oil
    - Low-fat milk or almond milk
    - Grated Parmesan cheese (optional)

- Salt and pepper to taste

- **Instructions**:
1.	Cook whole wheat pasta according to package instructions. Drain and set aside.
2. In a pan, sauté minced garlic in olive oil until fragrant.
3. Add sliced mushrooms and cook until tender.
4. Add fresh spinach leaves and cook until wilted.
5. Pour in low-fat milk (or almond milk) and simmer until the sauce thickens slightly.
6. Season with salt and pepper, then toss in the cooked pasta.
7.	Optionally, sprinkle grated Parmesan cheese on top before serving.

- **Benefits**: This recipe combines whole grains from whole wheat pasta with calcium-rich spinach and vitamin D from mushrooms. The low-fat milk provides additional calcium, while Parmesan cheese adds flavor and extra calcium.

2. **Grilled Salmon with Lemon Herb Quinoa:**

- **Ingredients**:
    - Salmon fillets
    - Quinoa
    - Fresh lemon juice
    - Freshly chopped herbs (such cilantro, dill, or parsley)
    - Olive oil
    - Salt and pepper

- **Instructions**:
    1. Cook quinoa according to package instructions and fluff with a fork. Stir in fresh lemon juice and chopped herbs.
    2. Preheat a grill or grill pan. Add salt and pepper to the salmon fillets after brushing them with olive oil.

    3. Grill salmon until cooked through and slightly charred on the edges.
    4. Serve grilled salmon over lemon herb quinoa.

- **Benefits**: This dish is rich in omega-3 fatty acids from salmon, which support bone health and reduce inflammation. Quinoa provides protein, calcium, magnesium, and fiber, while fresh herbs add antioxidants and flavor.

3. **Greek Yogurt Berry Smoothie Bowl:**

- **Ingredients**:
    - Greek yogurt (plain or flavored)
    - Mixed berries (strawberries, blueberries, raspberries)
    - Banana, sliced
    - Honey or maple syrup (optional)
    - Chopped nuts or granola as a garnish

- **Instructions**:
    1. In a blender, combine Greek yogurt, mixed berries, sliced banana, and honey or maple syrup if desired.
    2. Blend until smooth and creamy.
    3. Pour the smoothie into a bowl and top with granola or chopped nuts for added crunch.

- **Benefits**: Greek yogurt is high in calcium, protein, and probiotics that support bone health. Berries provide antioxidants, vitamins, and minerals, while bananas add potassium and fiber. Granola or nuts contribute healthy fats and additional nutrients.

These nutritious recipes are not only delicious but also packed with essential nutrients for stronger bones, making them ideal choices for individuals with osteoporosis or anyone looking to maintain optimal bone health.

Breakfast Ideas:

Having a nutritious breakfast is crucial for individuals with osteoporosis as it sets the tone for the day and provides essential nutrients for bone health. Here are some breakfast ideas specifically designed to support bone health and manage osteoporosis:

1. **Greek Yogurt Parfait**:
    - Ingredients: Greek yogurt (plain or flavored), mixed berries (strawberries,

blueberries, raspberries), granola, chia seeds, honey or maple syrup.

- Benefits: Greek yogurt is rich in calcium, protein, and probiotics that aid in bone strength. Berries provide antioxidants and vitamins, while chia seeds add omega-3s and fiber. Granola adds crunch and additional nutrients.

2. **Spinach and Mushroom Omelet**:

- Ingredients: Eggs, fresh spinach leaves, sliced mushrooms, onion, garlic, grated cheese (optional), olive oil, salt, and pepper.

- Benefits: Eggs offer vitamin D, protein, and minerals like phosphorus. Spinach provides calcium, magnesium, and vitamin K, while mushrooms add vitamin D. Cheese adds calcium and flavor.

3. **Oatmeal with Almond Butter and Banana:**

- Ingredients: Rolled oats, almond butter, banana slices, cinnamon, honey or maple syrup (optional), milk or almond milk.

- Benefits: Oats are a good source of fiber and minerals like magnesium and phosphorus. Almond butter adds healthy fats, calcium, and protein. Bananas provide potassium and vitamins.

4. **Avocado Toast with Smoked Salmon:**

- Ingredients: Whole grain bread, ripe avocado, smoked salmon slices, lemon juice, red pepper flakes (optional), salt, and pepper.

- Benefits: Whole grain bread offers fiber and nutrients. Avocado provides healthy fats, potassium, and vitamin K. Smoked salmon adds omega-3 fatty acids and protein.

5. **Chia Seed Pudding with Berries:**

- Ingredients: Chia seeds, almond milk, vanilla extract, mixed berries, honey or maple syrup (optional), sliced almonds or coconut flakes for topping.

- Benefits: Chia seeds are rich in omega-3s, fiber, calcium, and magnesium. Almond milk provides calcium and vitamin D. Berries offer antioxidants and vitamins.

6. **Smoothie Bowl with Spinach and Almond Milk:**

- Ingredients: Fresh spinach leaves, almond milk, banana, frozen berries, protein powder (optional), honey or maple syrup (optional), toppings like granola, nuts, or seeds.

- Benefits: Spinach adds calcium, magnesium, and vitamin K. Almond milk provides calcium and vitamin D. Berries offer antioxidants and flavor.

7. **Whole Grain Pancakes with Greek Yogurt and Fruit**:
    - Ingredients: Whole grain pancake mix, Greek yogurt, mixed fruit (such as berries, banana slices), honey or maple syrup.
    - Benefits: Whole grain pancakes offer fiber and nutrients. Greek yogurt adds calcium, protein, and probiotics. Fruit provides vitamins, antioxidants, and natural sweetness.

These breakfast ideas are nutrient-dense, balanced, and delicious, providing a variety of vitamins, minerals, and macronutrients essential for bone health and overall well-being. Pairing these breakfast options with regular physical activity and a healthy lifestyle can further support bone health and manage osteoporosis effectively.

Lunch and Dinner Recipes:

A balanced diet rich in nutrients essential for bone health can help slow down bone loss and improve bone density. Here are some lunch and dinner recipes that incorporate ingredients known to support bone health and may contribute to managing osteoporosis:

Lunch Ideas:

1. Salmon and Kale Salad:
   - **Ingredients**:
     - Grilled or baked salmon fillet
     - Fresh kale leaves, chopped
     - Cherry tomatoes, halved
     - Avocado, sliced
     - Red onion, thinly sliced
     - Walnuts or almonds, chopped
     - Olive oil
     - Lemon juice
     - Dijon mustard
     - Salt and pepper to taste

   Directions:
   1. In a large bowl, combine chopped kale, halved cherry tomatoes, sliced avocado, thinly sliced red onion, and chopped walnuts or almonds.
   2. Whisk together olive oil, lemon juice, Dijon mustard, salt, and pepper to make the dressing.
   3. Grill or bake salmon until cooked through and flake into chunks.
   4. Toss the salad with the dressing and top with salmon chunks before serving.

2. **Quinoa and Vegetable Stir-Fry**:

- **Ingredients**:
  - Cooked quinoa
  - Mixed vegetables (bell peppers, broccoli, carrots, snap peas)
  - Tofu or chicken breast strips
  - Garlic, minced
  - Ginger, grated
  - Soy sauce or tamari
  - Sesame oil
  - Sesame seeds
  - Green onions, chopped
  - Olive oil
  - Salt and pepper to taste

- **Directions**:

1. In a large skillet or wok, heat olive oil over medium-high heat. Add minced garlic and grated ginger, sauté until fragrant.

2. Add mixed vegetables and cook until slightly tender but still crisp.

3. Push the vegetables to the side of the skillet and add tofu or chicken strips. Cook until browned and cooked through.

4. Mix everything together and add cooked quinoa to the skillet.

5. Drizzle with soy sauce or tamari, sesame oil, and sprinkle with sesame seeds and chopped green onions before serving.

Dinner Ideas:

1. Spinach and Chickpea Curry:
   - **Ingredients**:
     - Cooked chickpeas
     - Fresh spinach leaves
     - Onion, diced
     - Garlic, minced
     - Ginger, grated
     - Tomatoes, diced
     - Coconut milk
     - Curry powder, turmeric, cumin, coriander
     - Olive oil
     - Fresh cilantro, chopped
     - Salt and pepper to taste

   - **Directions**:
     1. In a large saucepan, heat olive oil over medium heat. Add grated ginger, chopped garlic, and diced onion. Sauté until softened.
     2. Add diced tomatoes and cook until they start to break down.
     3. Stir in cooked chickpeas, curry powder, turmeric, cumin, coriander, salt, and pepper.
     4. Pour in coconut milk and let simmer for a few minutes.
     5. Add fresh spinach leaves and cook until wilted.

6. Garnish with chopped fresh cilantro before serving. Serve over brown rice or quinoa.

2. **Baked Herb-Crusted Chicken with Roasted Vegetables**:

- Ingredients:
  - Chicken breasts or thighs, boneless and skinless
  - Fresh herbs (rosemary, thyme, parsley), chopped
  - Garlic, minced
  - Lemon zest
  - Olive oil
  - Assorted vegetables (such as carrots, broccoli, cauliflower)
  - Salt and pepper to taste

- **Directions**:
1. Preheat oven to 375°F (190°C). Spread some olive oil on a baking dish.
2. In a bowl, mix chopped herbs, minced garlic, lemon zest, olive oil, salt, and pepper to create a marinade.
3. Coat chicken breasts or thighs with the herb marinade and place them in the baking dish.

4. Arrange assorted vegetables around the chicken in the baking dish. Sprinkle with salt, pepper, and a tiny bit of olive oil.

5. Bake in the preheated oven for about 25-30 minutes or until the chicken is cooked through and vegetables are tender.

These recipes are nutrient-dense and incorporate ingredients that support bone health, such as calcium-rich leafy greens, omega-3 fatty acids from salmon, protein from tofu or chicken, and various vegetables with vitamins and minerals. Incorporating these recipes into a balanced diet along with regular physical activity can contribute to managing osteoporosis and promoting overall well-being. Adjust the recipes based on personal preferences and dietary needs.

Snacks and Beverages:

Snacks and beverages play a significant role in supporting bone health and managing osteoporosis by providing essential nutrients such as calcium, vitamin D, magnesium, and protein. Here are some snack ideas and beverages that can help in the fight against osteoporosis:

Snacks:

1. Greek Yogurt with Berries:
   - Greek yogurt is high in calcium and protein, which are beneficial for bone health. Add a handful of berries for antioxidants and flavor.

2. Almonds or Walnuts:
   - Nuts like almonds and walnuts are rich in calcium, magnesium, and healthy fats. They provide a filling and healthy snack.

3. Hummus with Veggie Sticks:
   - Hummus, made from chickpeas, provides calcium and protein. Pair it with carrot sticks, cucumber slices, or bell pepper strips for added vitamins and minerals.

4. Cheese and Whole Grain Crackers:
   - Cheese is a good source of calcium and protein. Choose whole grain crackers for fiber and nutrients.

5. Hard-Boiled Eggs:
   - Eggs are rich in vitamin D and protein, which are beneficial for bone health. A hard-boiled egg makes for a convenient and nutritious snack.

6. Cottage Cheese with Fruit:

- Cottage cheese is high in protein and calcium. Serve it with fresh fruits like berries, pineapple, or peaches for added vitamins and flavor.

7. Edamame:

- Edamame (young soybeans) are a good source of calcium, magnesium, and protein. They can be enjoyed steamed and lightly salted.

Beverages:

1. Milk or Fortified Plant-Based Milk:

- Milk is a classic source of calcium and vitamin D. Choose low-fat or fortified plant-based milk options like almond milk, soy milk, or oat milk for those who are lactose intolerant or prefer non-dairy alternatives.

2. Calcium-Fortified Orange Juice:

- Many brands offer calcium-fortified orange juice, providing an easy way to increase calcium intake. Look for options with added vitamin D for better absorption.

3. Green Smoothies:

- Blend leafy greens like kale or spinach with fruits, Greek yogurt or plant-based protein powder, and almond milk for a nutrient-packed beverage high in calcium, vitamin K, and antioxidants.

4. Herbal Teas:

- Herbal teas such as chamomile, peppermint, or ginger can be soothing and hydrating options. Some herbal teas also contain minerals like magnesium that contribute to bone health.

5. Bone Broth:

- Homemade or store-bought bone broth is rich in minerals like calcium, magnesium, and phosphorus, which are beneficial for bone strength. It can be consumed as a warm beverage or used as a base for soups and stews.

6. Smoothies with Nutritional Boosters:

- Enhance smoothies with calcium-rich ingredients like yogurt, almond butter, chia seeds, and leafy greens. Adding a scoop of protein powder or collagen peptides can also support bone health.

7. Water with Lemon or Cucumber:
   - Staying hydrated is critical to general health, including bone health. Infuse water with slices of lemon or cucumber for a refreshing and hydrating drink.

Incorporating these snacks and beverages into a balanced diet, along with regular physical activity and other lifestyle measures, can contribute to better bone health and help manage osteoporosis. It's essential to choose nutrient-dense options and consider individual dietary preferences and needs.

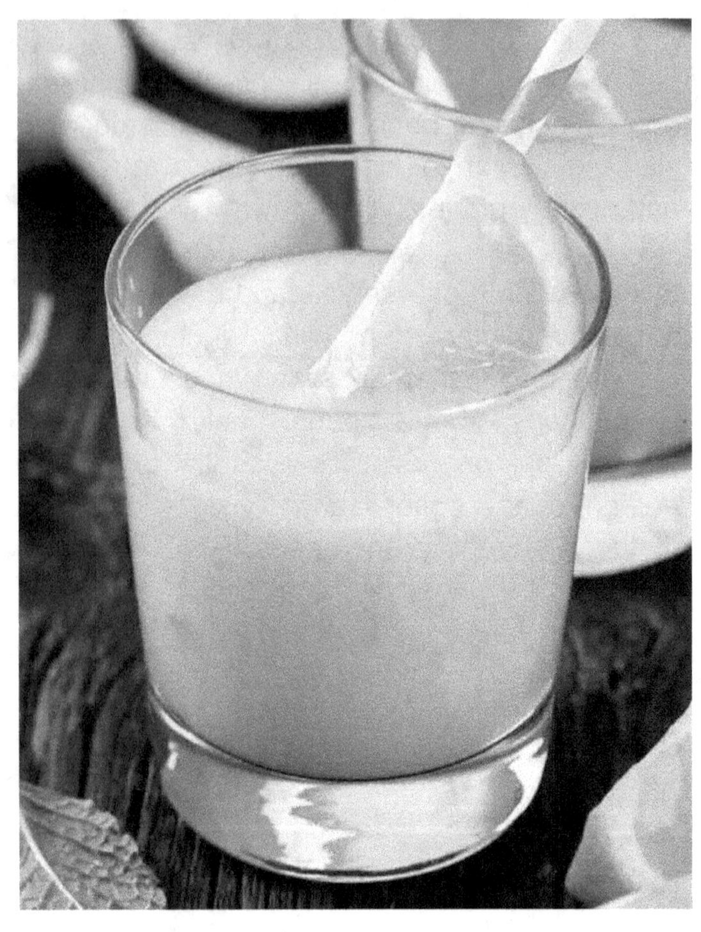

Conclusion

In conclusion, achieving long-term bone health and effectively managing osteoporosis requires a holistic approach that includes monitoring progress and making sustainable lifestyle changes. Regular monitoring of bone density through follow-up bone density tests and consultations with healthcare professionals is crucial to track progress and make informed decisions about treatment and lifestyle adjustments.

Additionally, adopting sustainable lifestyle changes is key to maintaining optimal bone health over time. This includes incorporating a balanced diet rich in calcium, vitamin D, magnesium, and other essential nutrients for bone strength. Regular physical activity, especially weight-bearing exercises and resistance training, helps to build and maintain bone density. Avoiding smoking and excessive alcohol intake is also crucial because they can harm bone health.

Furthermore, practicing stress reduction techniques, getting adequate sleep, and managing chronic conditions that affect bone health contribute to overall well-being and long-term bone health. It's essential to prioritize self-care and make health-conscious choices to support bone strength and prevent fractures associated with osteoporosis.

Long-term management of osteoporosis and preservation of strong, healthy bones throughout life can be attained by individuals through a proactive approach to bone health, consistent monitoring, and sustainable lifestyle modifications.